RENAL SYSTEM

Renal System

Brian A. Jackson, Ph.D.

Professor
Department of Physiology
University of Kentucky
  College of Medicine
Lexington, Kentucky

Cobern E. Ott, Ph.D.

Professor
Department of Physiology
University of Kentucky
  College of Medicine
Lexington, Kentucky

**Fence Creek
Publishing**

**Madison,
Connecticut**

Typesetter: Pagesetters, Brattleboro, VT
Printer: Port City Press, Baltimore, MD
Illustrations by Visible Productions, Fort Collins, CO
Distributors:

United States and Canada
Blackwell Science, Inc.
Commerce Place
350 Main Street
Malden, MA 02148
Telephone orders: 800-215-1000 or 781-388-8250
Fax orders: 781-388-8270

Australia
Blackwell Science, PTY LTD.
54 University Street
Carlton, Victoria 3053
Telephone orders: 61-39-347-0300
Fax orders: 61-39-347-5001

Outside North America and Australia
Blackwell Science, LTD.
c/o Marston Book Service, LTD.
P.O. Box 269
Abingdon Oxon, OX 14 4XN England
Telephone orders: 44-1-235-465500
Fax orders: 44-1-235-465555

1 2 3 4 5 6 7 8 9 10

TABLE OF CONTENTS

PREFACE

It has been our experience that students at all levels find renal function one of the most difficult physiological systems to comprehend. There is no question that the kidney is considerably more conceptual than most organ systems. In addition, the quantitative nature of many of these concepts can be confusing. Therefore, based on our collective teaching experiences to date, we have attempted to develop a textbook that will make the kidney less intimidating and therefore more understandable, particularly for medical students.

Chapter 1 introduces the reader to the concept of body fluid homeostasis and emphasizes the critical role that the kidneys play in this process. As a preface to a description of the major body fluid compartments, we provide a comprehensive review of fundamental chemical and physical concepts that are critical to the understanding of renal function. Chapter 2 presents an overview of renal anatomy, provides an appreciation of the magnitude of overall renal function, and introduces the key components of renal function including glomerular filtration, tubular reabsorption, and tubular secretion. Chapters 3 and 4 focus on the regulation of glomerular filtration and renal tubular reabsorption and secretion, respectively. With this fundamental information in hand, the remainder of the book emphasizes the role of the kidney in water and sodium chloride homeostasis (Chapter 5), potassium, calcium, and phosphate homeostasis (Chapter 6), and acid–base homeostasis (Chapter 7).

Although the fundamental content is similar to that of several excellent texts that are already available, we have incorporated several unique aspects into this new book. First, we have purposely avoided unnecessary detail. For example, a solid appreciation of glomerular filtration does not require a detailed analysis of filtration pressure equilibrium and disequilibrium. Similarly, we believe that at this level, it is not necessary to describe in a step-by-step fashion the nuances of the so-called "single effect" in the countercurrent multiplication system. In our experience, this level of detail actually detracts from the student's ability to understand the fundamental and most important aspects of renal function.

Second, whenever possible we have attempted to consider renal function in an applied setting. For example, why and how does glomerular filtration change in response to hemorrhage or dehydration? What are the implications of diuretic therapy for renal medullary tonicity and renal concentrating ability? In keeping with the integrative nature of this series of textbooks, we have also emphasized the similarities as well as the unique differences between the kidney and other organ systems. For example, we compare and contrast the driving forces for fluid movement across glomerular and systemic capillaries. This integrative theme is particularly emphasized in discussions of ion homeostasis. For example, we have stressed that the maintenance of calcium or hydrogen ion homeostasis is dependent on the coordinated responses of several organ systems in addition to the kidney.

Finally, in order to facilitate and reinforce the learning process, each chapter contains the presentation and resolution of a short clinical case and also offers a series of multiple choice questions complete with answers and explanations.

Brian A. Jackson, Ph.D. and Cobern E. Ott, Ph.D.

ACKNOWLEDGMENTS

The authors would like to thank Mr. Matt Harris of Fence Creek Publishing for the opportunity to write this textbook, and for his patience and encouragement throughout the writing process. We would also like to thank Ms. Jane Edwards for her expert editorial assistance.

This book is dedicated to my wife Jean and my son Marc
for their understanding during the writing process when more time
was spent with the word processor than with them.

This book is dedicated to my wife Sue Helen
for her continuous support and infinite patience.

INTRODUCTION

Renal System is one of eight titles in the *Integrated Medical Sciences (IMS) Series* from Fence Creek Publishing. These books have been designed as course supplements and aids for board review for first- and second-year medical students. Rather than focusing on the individual basic science disciplines, the books in the *IMS Series* have been designed to highlight the points of integration between the sciences, including clinical correlations where appropriate. Each chapter begins with a clinical case, the resolution of which requires the application of basic science concepts to clinical problems. Extensive use of margin notes, figures, tables, and questions illuminates core biomedical concepts with which medical students often have difficulty.

Each book in the *IMS Series* shares common features and formats. Attempts have been made to present difficult concepts in a brief and focused format and to provide a pedagogical aid that facilitates both knowledge acquisition and also review.

Given the long gestation period necessary to publish a book, it is often impossible for publishers to keep pace with the changes and advances that occur so rapidly. However, the authors and the publisher recognize the need to have access to the most current information and are committed to keeping *Renal System* as up to date as possible between editions. As the field of renal physiology evolves, updates to this text may be posted on our web site periodically at http://www.fencecreek.com.

We hope that the student finds the format and the text material relevant, interesting, and challenging. The authors, as well as the Fence Creek staff, welcome your comments and suggestions for use in future editions.

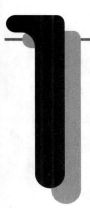

BODY FLUID HOMEOSTASIS

CHAPTER OUTLINE

INTRODUCTION OF CLINICAL CASES

Case 1: Volume Disturbance and Normal Renal Function

A 70-year-old woman from a small town was admitted to the local hospital after having been found in her house unconscious. Her medical history was obtained from friends who stated that she had been well until 3 years ago when she suffered a stroke, fell, and broke her hip. After a long hospitalization, she recovered enough to return home. She had not been seen by her friends for several days when she was found. Her blood pressure was 105 mm Hg systolic and 60 mm Hg diastolic. Her heart rate was 115 beats/min. Her lips and mouth were covered with dry secretions, and her skin elasticity was poor. She was disoriented and unable to answer questions. Laboratory results are given in Table 1-1. A urine sample was not available.

Case 2: Abnormal Renal Function

A 30-year-old woman developed a sore throat followed 2 weeks later by hematuria (blood in the urine) and generalized edema (fluid accumulation in tissues). Six weeks later, she noticed that her urine had a reddish-brown tinge. Her physician determined that she was mildly hypertensive with a blood pressure of 140 mm Hg systolic and 96 mm Hg diastolic, and that the urine contained numerous red blood cells (RBCs). She excreted 3.5 g of protein a day (proteinuria), and her blood urea nitrogen (BUN) was 40 mg/100 mL. At this point, the diagnosis of glomerulonephritis was made. Over the next 8 years she had increasing hypertension, proteinuria, and developed renal failure. In the past year, she had had problems with headaches, nosebleeds, vomiting, and general weakness. There was swelling of the ankles and puffiness around her eyes. Because of the increasing severity of the symptoms, she presented to the emergency department and was subsequently admitted to the hospital. She was somewhat lethargic and obviously ill. Her blood pressure was 230/120 mm Hg, her pulse rate was 120/min, and her temperature was 101°F. During the first 24 hours of observation, she passed 300 mL of urine. A venous blood sample gave the following data, which are summarized in Table 1-2.

TABLE 1-1 ▶

Laboratory Data from a Panel of Tests Measuring Seven Variables

Test	Result
Plasma	
Blood urea nitrogen	120 mg/100 mL (increased)[a]
Creatinine	4.0 mg/100 mL (increased)
Sodium	170 mEq/L (increased)
Potassium	4.1 mEq/L (normal)
Chloride	132 mEq/L (increased)
Bicarbonate	25 mEq/L (normal)
Glucose	90 mg/100 mL (normal)
Urine	
Not available	

[a] Increased indicates a value higher than normal.

TABLE 1-2 ▶

Results of Venous Blood Sample

Test	Result
Blood urea nitrogen	176 mg/dL (very high)
Creatinine	14 mg/dL (very high)
Sodium	131 mEq/L (low)
Potassium	6.2 mEq/L (high)
Bicarbonate	16 mmol/L (low)
Calcium	7.4 mg/dL (low)
Albumin	2.9 g/dL (low)
Hematocrit	18% (very low)

HOMEOSTASIS

Normal Renal Function

*The **major function of the kidney** is to keep the volume and composition of the body fluid compartments constant.*

In the simplest terms, the function of the kidneys is to preserve whole body fluid homeostasis by maintaining a constant volume and composition of the body fluid compartments. Although simple in concept, the inability of the kidneys to perform their function leads to many complex and identifiable abnormalities. The normal function of the kidney and the consequences of renal failure may be appreciated best by the close examination of a patient with end-stage renal failure given in Case 2 above. This case will be used to discuss specific aspects of abnormal renal function. In addition, a very small list of normal plasma values is given later in the chapter. In examining a complex situation, whether it involves a patient or an experimental animal protocol, an idea of whether a plasma sodium (Na^+) concentration of 130 milliequivalents/liter (mEq/L) or a plasma potassium (K^+) concentration of 7 mEq/L is meaningful must be appreciated.

To appreciate the role of the kidneys, the clinical history must be considered as well as the laboratory results. First, the patient presented above (Case 2) is hypertensive. This could result from the retention of too much salt and water in the plasma or from excess formation of vasoconstrictor substances, such as angiotensin II. Because the kidney is responsible for the control of both functions, the hypertensive situation may be the result of both. Second, the patient also has an accumulation of fluid in her extremities, which manifests as edema. The major force for retaining fluid in the cardiovascular compartment is the colloid osmotic pressure, which is, in part, a direct function of the plasma albumin concentration. Because the patient's plasma albumin concentration is approximately half normal, it is not surprising that there is movement of fluid from the cardiovascular system into the interstitial space, which results in the edema. It should be emphasized that it is not the kidney's role to regulate the plasma albumin concentration; that is a function of the liver. However, one frequent hallmark of many forms of renal disease is the abnormal loss of protein into the urine. Thus, the inability of the kidney to prevent the loss of protein in the urine results in a change in the distribution of volume in the body fluid compartments. Although many times it is one of the last clinical symptoms to be appreciated, renal failure also often results in a very low hematocrit. The above patient has a hematocrit of less than 50% of normal. The kidney secretes erythropoietin, which stimulates RBC production by the bone marrow. In the absence of functional renal tissue, the amount of erythropoietin secreted decreases, and RBC production declines. The kidney again has control over the body fluid volumes. In this case, it is the RBC volume in the cardiovascular system.

A quick perusal of the laboratory values above for Case 2 reveals many other abnormalities in whole body fluid homeostasis. Urea is the result of protein metabolism and is measured as the nitrogen associated with urea in the blood; that is, BUN. Creatinine is derived from muscle metabolism as a by-product of phosphocreatine. The important concept is that both are metabolic waste products and can be used as an index of other metabolic waste products in the plasma. A major role of the kidney is to remove them from the circulation. In the presence of a failing kidney, the metabolic waste products simply increase in the plasma and alter the composition of the extracellular fluid (ECF).

There are also several electrolyte disturbances. The plasma Na^+ concentration is low. It is a common mistake to think that a low Na^+ concentration is the result of a Na^+ deficiency when, in fact, an excess of water is just as likely to be the cause. In this case, the patient is excreting only 300 mL a day of fluid as urine. Thus, retention of water results in increased volume and a decrease in the plasma Na^+ concentration, both of which represent another example of alterations in the volume and composition of the body fluid compartments. This alteration in volume may have clinical consequences. Although Na^+ is important for the generation of action potentials, it is much more important for the regulation of water movement into and out of the cells. Because Na^+ is the major cation in the ECF, it plays a large role in dictating the extracellular osmolarity, which will be discussed in greater detail later in this chapter. The consequence of the low Na^+ concentration is the movement of water into all the cells. When water moves into brain cells, the cells swell. However, the skull is nonelastic, and the increased cellular volume may compress the blood vessels that supply the brain. The resulting decreased blood flow can have serious neurologic consequences. A major concern with low Na^+ concentration in the blood (i.e., hyponatremia) or high Na^+ concentration in the blood (i.e., hypernatremia) is movement of water into and out of the brain cells.

The plasma K^+ concentration is increased. Another role for the kidney is to excrete K^+. In the absence of the ability to excrete K^+, the plasma concentration of K^+ increases. Extracellular K^+ is the prime determinant of the resting membrane potential. An increase in extracellular K^+ leads to the development of spontaneous depolarization as a result of an increased resting membrane potential and may in fact lead to cardiac fibrillation and death.

The bicarbonate (HCO_3^-) concentration is low. Although an accurate acid–base diagnosis can be made only from analysis of an arterial blood sample, the decreased base concentration reflected by the HCO_3^- suggests an acidotic condition. The kidney normally excretes hydrogen (H^+) and synthesizes HCO_3^-. An inability to do both results in acidosis. Because an optimal pH is necessary for the proper function of many intracellular enzymes, it is easy to see how an acid–base disturbance could have many undesirable effects on the body.

The decreased calcium (Ca^{2+}) concentration is another aspect of diminished renal function. The kidney is responsible for the conservation of Ca^{2+} and for converting inactive 25-hydroxyvitamin D_3 to the active form of 1,25-dihydroxyvitamin D_3. The 1,25-dihydroxyvitamin D_3 is necessary for Ca^{2+} uptake by the intestine. The lowered Ca^{2+} concentration has both short-term and long-term consequences. In the short term, the decreased Ca^{2+} may lead to muscle tetany; in the long term, the low Ca^{2+} stimulates parathyroid hormone (PTH) and results in bone resorption. Before the discovery and synthesis of 1,25-dihydroxyvitamin D_3, a major clinical problem with chronic renal failure was the loss of bone mass and frequent fractures.

Thus, it can be seen that the kidney has many regulatory functions, including at least the following:

- Regulation of the osmolarity and volume of the body fluid compartments
- Regulation of electrolyte balance
- Regulation of acid–base balance
- Excretion of metabolic by-products and foreign substances
- Production, secretion, and activation of hormones

Chronic renal failure often results in many physical abnormalities, such as edema and hypertension, as well as abnormalities in body fluid volumes and composition.

In summary, it is simple to state that the function of the kidneys is to maintain constant volume and composition of the body fluid compartments. However, the constancy of the volume and composition of the body fluid compartments has important consequences for normal function of many of the other systems of the body, including, but not limited to, the cardiovascular, muscular, and nervous systems. One thing to be noted is that chronic renal failure may not be readily recognized from physical symptoms. A physician who makes a diagnosis of hypertension may be tempted to first look for a cardiovascular problem. Edema may be thought to be a problem with congestive heart failure (CHF), whereas vomiting might be considered a problem with the gastrointestinal (GI) system. The surest way to identify a renal problem is to measure the build-up of nitrogenous waste products in the blood, in particular, creatinine.

Homeostasis and Dynamic Equilibrium

Homeostasis is the maintenance of the stability of the body's internal environment. Dynamic equilibrium is the balance between input and output that keeps the internal environment stable.

The term *homeostasis* has been used frequently to indicate a state of "standing still," which is another way of saying that things do not change. That is absolutely correct. For instance, in a healthy individual, the plasma volume is maintained nearly constant by a tremendous number of physiologic control systems that are designed to regulate that volume. However, the body fluid compartments are in a continuous state of flux. To appreciate renal function, it must be understood that what is maintained is determined by the difference between what goes in and what comes out. The relationship between input and output is illustrated in Fig. 1-1. One concept that must be emphasized is that the kidney cannot manufacture fluid, it can only decrease the continued loss. It is a common misconception that a decrease in urine output, for example, increases body fluid volumes. This is not so; it only diminishes any further loss.

Physiologic feedback systems are the mechanisms that maintain internal stability. A change in one controlled variable invokes feedback mechanisms that act in the opposite (negative) direction to return the controlled variable toward the normal value.

Rather than using the mechanical analogy above, the control system can be replaced by the physiologic feedback system shown in Fig. 1-2. In this relationship, volume is still the controlled variable. In a negative feedback system, a change in one variable elicits a response in the opposite (negative) direction to oppose the change. If the plasma volume decreases, the decrease in plasma volume leads to an increase in water intake and thus an increase in volume. The decreased plasma volume also increases the renal reabsorption of water, which helps to maintain plasma volume. The relationship between decreased plasma volume and increased water intake is complex and involves many neural components. As will be discussed in later chapters, the relationship between decreased plasma volume and increased water reabsorption is also very complex and involves several underlying and additional control systems. However, the homeostatic mechanisms of the body operate, in this case, to maintain the plasma volume. Exactly the opposite occurs if plasma volume is increased. Also, a change in either intake or output can change the plasma volume. An increase in water intake in the presence of an

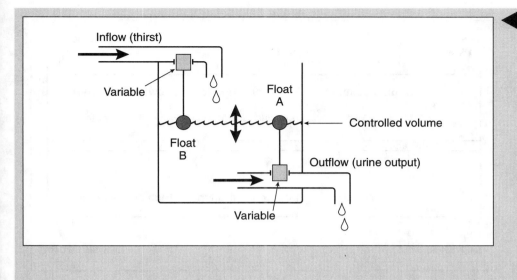

FIGURE 1-1
Mechanical Control System to Maintain Constant Tank Volume. The floats are the control systems that maintain constant volume by regulating input as well as output. If volume tends to go up for some reason, the water level in the tank increases, and float A rises, which allows more outflow to return the volume in the tank to a constant level. Float B also rises to decrease intake. If the water level goes down, float A falls and decreases output while float B falls to increase input until the volume is returned to normal. The volume is maintained constant, and the tank volume is in a state of homeostasis; that is, it changes very little over the long term. Although the volume maintained is relatively stable, the water in the tank now is not necessarily the same water that was in the tank a few hours ago. Thus homeostasis, a stable volume, is maintained by a dynamic equilibrium between input and output.

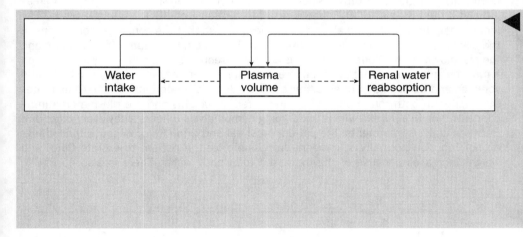

FIGURE 1-2
Physiologic Control System to Maintain Constant Plasma Volume. In this and all subsequent, similar diagrams, a solid line represents a direct relationship, whereas a dashed line represents an inverse relationship. Thus, the system A → B --> C means that as A increases, then B also increases; or, as A decreases, then B decreases. Conversely, if B increases, then C decreases, and vice versa. This system uses negative feedback actions and emphasizes the relationships and the interrelationships among the variables. Changes in plasma volume affect both intake and output to maintain a normal plasma volume.

unchanged water reabsorption can lead to increased volume. Conversely, an increase in water reabsorption in the presence of an unchanged intake can also lead to an increased volume.

What happens when the kidney fails? The patient must still ingest food and drink fluids, but one part of the dynamic equilibrium system does not work; that is, the regulated output is gone. The volume in the tank or the plasma volume cannot increase forever. There are only two options. Either a new output system must be created by renal transplantation or some artificial means must be used to substitute for the kidney. In fact, most patients with severe renal failure are kept alive by artificial means.

ARTIFICIAL HOMEOSTASIS

Hemodialysis is a technique that uses an artificial kidney to treat many patients with chronic renal failure. However, many changes in body fluid volumes and composition occur between treatments. A very simplified diagram of an artificial kidney is illustrated in Fig. 1-3. During dialysis, blood from the patient's artery is routed to one side of a semipermeable artificial membrane and returned to the body via a vein. Dialysis fluid, similar to a modified balanced salt solution, flows on the other side of the membrane. The artificial membrane is impermeable to large molecules, proteins, and RBCs. There is a positive hydrostatic pressure from the blood to the dialysis fluid, and thus, water is filtered by the hydrostatic pressure difference across the membrane to remove it from the body. Small molecules diffuse across the membrane according to the concentration

FIGURE 1-3 ▶

Diagrammatic Representation of an Artificial Kidney. *Water is filtered from the blood by hydrostatic pressure. Small molecules diffuse down their concentration gradient.*

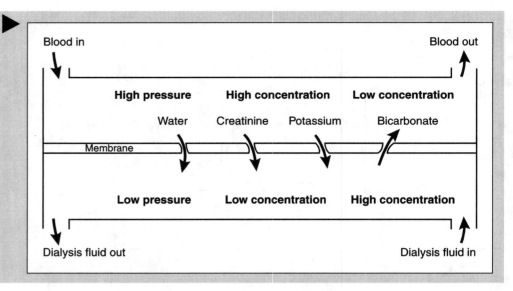

differences between the blood and dialysis fluid. For example, during renal failure the plasma K^+ concentration increases, and the plasma HCO_3^- concentration decreases. During dialysis, then, K^+ diffuses out of the blood into a dialysis fluid low in K^+, whereas a dialysis fluid high in HCO_3^- would result in diffusion of HCO_3^- into the blood. The ionic concentration of the dialysis fluid is designed so that the concentration of ions in the plasma is near normal following treatment. Thus, both the volume of body water and the plasma concentrations of many ions can be corrected during hemodialysis. However, it must be emphasized that this is an intermittent intervention, and changes in body fluid volumes and composition often occur between dialysis treatments. Fig. 1-4 illustrates the change in both total body water (illustrated as weight) and the plasma creatinine concentration in a patient who is undergoing hemodialysis 6 hours a day every other day. Between dialysis treatments, the patient must eat and drink fluid. Because the kidneys do not function normally, it is nearly impossible for the patient to excrete fluid, and weight increases because of the increased total body water. There is also no way to

Between hemodialysis treatments, body fluid volumes and composition change. They can be restored toward normal by hemodialysis treatment.

FIGURE 1-4 ▶

Changes in Body Weight and Plasma Creatinine Concentration with Time in a Patient Undergoing Intermittent Hemodialysis. *Between treatments, water retention occurs, and weight increases. Continued metabolism results in increased plasma creatinine concentration. During treatment, both body water (A) and plasma creatinine concentration (B) are returned toward normal.*

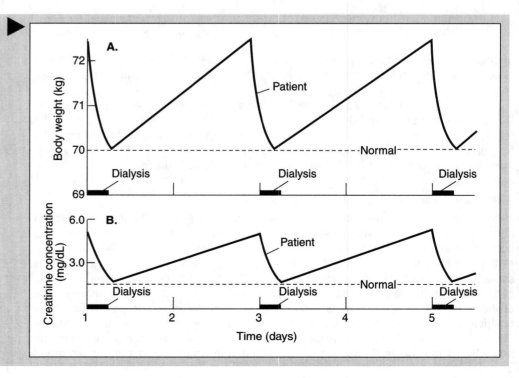

excrete the creatinine that is continuously generated from muscle metabolism, so the plasma concentration of creatinine increases. During dialysis, water is removed by filtration across the membrane, and weight decreases. Similarly, creatinine diffuses from the high concentration in blood to the dialysis fluid, and the creatinine concentration in the plasma also decreases. It can be appreciated that total body water and the creatinine concentration can be decreased during dialysis, but there are fluctuations in both on a day-to-day basis. Obviously, similar changes can occur in many electrolytes that may be corrected during dialysis, but they also change between dialysis sessions. The physician attempts to do in 6 hours every 2 days what the kidney does 24 hours a day, 7 days a week. Life is preserved, but homeostasis suffers.

Recent advances have allowed the use of chronic peritoneal dialysis to replace the external artificial kidney in a number of patients. With this technique, dialysis fluid is placed in the abdominal cavity and allowed to equilibrate over time with the ECF. After several hours, the fluid is removed and replaced with fresh dialysis fluid. Although this procedure obviates many of the large changes that occur between hemodialysis treatments and allows the patient to travel during dialysis, the fluid must be exchanged several times a day. In addition, the efficiency of the technique is limited by the volume of fluid used and the frequency of exchange. The increased risk of infection and resulting peritonitis is also a concern.

REVIEW OF CHEMICAL AND PHYSICAL CONCEPTS

Even in subjects with healthy kidneys, there can be disturbances in fluid volumes and composition that might occur, for example, during dehydration, excess salt intake, or hormonal dysfunction. Although this text is primarily concerned with renal function, many students have difficulty understanding renal function without a solid grasp of many physical and chemical concepts. Thus, a rather large section of this chapter is devoted to these concepts before proceeding to renal regulation. In addition to understanding fundamental renal function, a clear understanding of the normal volumes and concentrations is critical for the successful management of fluid and electrolyte disorders.

Common Chemical Units

The composition of the body fluid compartments is expressed in many different units. Many of the units used are simply the victims of history, but remain today. For instance, the concentration of glucose is still given mostly in units of milligrams% (mg%) or milligrams/deciliter (mg/dL), although some clinical laboratories report the units in millimoles/liter (mmol/L). Many plasma electrolytes are measured as mEq/L or mmol/L, whereas total solute concentration is measured in milliosmoles (mOsm)/kg H_2O or mOsm/L. Ca^{2+} is even more troublesome and is expressed in many different ways, including mg%, mmol/L, or mEq/L, and all three units result in different numerical values. A normal plasma Ca^{2+} value may be reported as 1.2 mmol/L, 2.4 mEq/L, or 4.8 mg/dL, all of which represent the same concentration. It is also of utmost importance to be able to convert between different units. Suppose it is determined that a severely acidotic patient requires 120 mEq of HCO_3^- to raise his plasma HCO_3^- concentration from 10 mEq/L to 20 mEq/L, but the only available HCO_3^- is in 50-mL vials containing a 7.5% solution of sodium bicarbonate ($NaHCO_3$). How much must be given?

Historically, the most common chemical unit is the term percent (%). It is simply a measure of mass/volume and, with no qualifier, a simple percent means grams/100 mL. Because many physiologic concentrations are dilute, the mg% unit is often used and implies mg/100 mL. As an example, normal plasma glucose concentration is approximately 80 mg% or 80 mg of glucose per 100 mL of plasma. In many instances, it is common to substitute mg/dL for mg%. Because a deciliter is one tenth of a liter (i.e., 100 mL), mg% and mg/dL are identical. Another common unit is vol%. This implies volume/100 mL of solution. The concentration of oxygen in arterial blood is approximately

> The abbreviation **mg%** means **mg/100 mL of solution** and is the same unit as **mg/dL**.

20 vol%, which means that there are 20 mL of oxygen dissolved in every 100 mL of blood.

Many substances in physiology are measured by simple concentration. A mmol/L of any compound is simply the number of millimoles/liter of solution. Because the molecular weight of Na^+ is 23, and the molecular weight of chloride (Cl^-) is 35.5, 1 mmol of NaCl would weigh 58.5 mg. If 58.5 mg of NaCl is dissolved in 1 L of solution, the concentration is 1 mmol/L. A mmol/L concentration is many times abbreviated as mM. If 117 mg of NaCl were dissolved in 1 L, the concentration would be 2 mmol/L. Obviously, the heavier the substance, the more mass is required for the same concentration. A 1 mmol/L solution of Ca^{2+}, with a molecular weight of 40, would require 40 mg/L, whereas Na^+, with a molecular weight of 23, would require only 23 mg/L.

Most electrolytes in plasma are dissociated and carry a charge when in solution. Their concentration is often measured in mEq/L, which is a measure of charge concentration, and it is the charge on the molecules that determines electrical activity in the body. For example, the difference between intracellular K^+ concentration and extracellular K^+ concentration determines the resting membrane potential, and it is the positive charge on the K^+ molecule that determines the electrical potential difference across the membrane. Similarly, it is movement of the positive charge on the Na^+ that initiates the action potential. Some molecules have multiple charges. Calcium exists in solution as Ca^{2+}, whereas iron may exist as Fe^{3+}. The total number of mEq of an ion in 1 L of solution is a function of the millimolar concentration of the ion and the charge on the ion. To determine the mEq/L concentration of any ion, the concentration of the ion is multiplied by the charge on the ion. For instance, a 2 mmol/L solution of Ca^{2+} has a concentration of 4 mEq/L (2 mmol/L $\times$ 2 charges/ion). It must be emphasized that milliequivalents can be determined only for individual ions. A 1 mmol/L solution of $CaCl_2$ dissolves into Ca^{2+} + Cl^- + Cl^-. There would be 2 mEq/L of Ca^{2+} (1 mmol/L $\times$ 2 charges/ion) and 2 mEq/L of Cl^- (2 mmol/L $\times$ 1 charge/ion). Because the number of positive milliequivalents and the number of negative milliequivalents are equal, the solution is electrically neutral. In the body, it is the separation of charges that give rise to electrical potentials.

Although separation of charge can give rise to electrical voltage differences, the separation of the total number of particles can give rise to osmotic pressure differences. The total solute concentration is measured in mOsm/L. To be precise, it is actually measured as mOsm/kg H_2O as a carry over from physical chemistry. However, because physiologic solutions are relatively dilute, the terms are often used interchangeably both in the clinics and in research. The importance of osmotic concentration in the regulation of body fluid volumes is that small differences in osmotic pressure across cell membranes cause water to move as a result of osmosis. As shown in Fig. 1-5, a difference in 1 mOsm/L creates a pressure of 19.6 mm Hg to cause water to move from the area of lower osmotic pressure to higher osmotic pressure. The osmotic concentration on both sides of the membrane is relatively high, but it is the difference in osmotic concentration that is important. It would require a hydrostatic pressure of 19.6 mm Hg in the opposite direction to prevent the water movement as a result of the 1 mOsm/L osmotic concentration difference. The pressure generated by the difference in osmotic concentration is often referred to as the osmotic pressure. It is not dependent on the size or the charge of the particle. One large protein molecule with a negative charge exerts the same osmotic pressure as one small Ca^{2+} molecule with two positive charges.

Often, osmolarity is referenced to plasma. A solution with the same osmolarity as plasma is said to be isotonic, whereas any solution with an osmolarity greater than plasma is said to be hypertonic. Similarly, a solution with an osmolarity less than plasma is labeled as hypotonic. This distinction is small but sometimes important. A solution of 1200 mOsm/L is iso-osmotic to a urine sample with a concentration of 1200 mOsm/L, but both are hypertonic relative to plasma. Conversely, a urine sample with a concentration of 100 mOsm/L is hypotonic to plasma but is iso-osmotic to a 100 mOsm/L solution.

The osmolarity of any solution can be measured in the laboratory and also can be approximated if one knows the concentration of particles in the solution. It is a simple calculation to multiply the concentration by the number of particles. This is particularly useful in a clinical situation if the measured osmolarity is unavailable. If there are multiple molecules, they all must be taken into account because the effects of all particles are additive. Consider a solution that has a 1 mmol/L concentration of $CaCl_2$

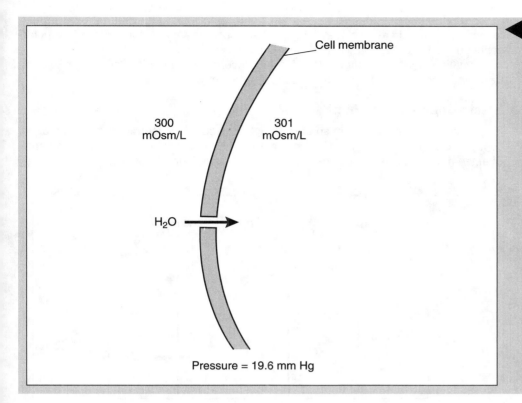

Small Differences in Osmolarity across a Cell Membrane Result in Water Movement from Lower Osmolarity to Higher Osmolarity. The osmolarity on both sides of the membrane is high, but the 1 mOsm/L difference creates a large ($\cong$ 19.6 mm Hg) pressure gradient for water to move.

and a 2 mmol/L concentration of NaCl. In solution, the $CaCl_2$ dissolves into three particles: $Ca^{2+} + Cl^- + Cl^-$. Thus, each millimole of $CaCl_2$ contributes 3 milliosmoles. The NaCl dissolves into two particles: $Na^+ + Cl^-$. The NaCl contributes two particles per millimole and, because there are 2 millimoles, it contributes 4 milliosmoles. The total osmolarity of the solution is the sum of both, or 7 mOsm/L.

Common Chemical Example

Perhaps the easiest way to explain the interrelationships among the various physical properties is to use a common example of a 22.2 mg% or 22.2 mg/dL solution of $CaCl_2$.

Using mg% or mg/dL. As stated earlier, mg% and mg/dL are the same units. A 22.2 mg% and a 22.2 mg/dL solution of $CaCl_2$ both have 22.2 mg of $CaCl_2$ for every 100 mL (or deciliter) of solution. This is equivalent to 222 mg/L.

Using mmol/L. To determine millimolar concentration, divide the amount by the molecular weight. The molecular weight of Ca^{2+} is 40, and the molecular weight of Cl^- is 35.5; therefore, 1 mmol of $CaCl_2$ weighs 111 mg [$Ca^{2+} = 40 + 2 \times (Cl^- = 35.5)$]. Thus, a 222 mg/L solution of $CaCl_2$ would contain 2 mmol/L; that is, (222 mg/L)/(111 mg/millimole). It should be intuitively obvious that the amount of any compound can be determined by the reverse process. Simply multiply the millimolar concentration by the molecular weight and take into account the difference in volume between liters and deciliters if necessary.

Using mEq/L. To determine the milliequivalent concentration of any ion, multiply the total millimolar concentration of that ion by the charge on the ion. Each mmol/L $CaCl_2$ in solution dissolves into $Ca^{2+} + Cl^- + Cl^-$. Because the concentration of Ca^{2+} is 2 mmol/L, and the charge on the Ca^{2+} is two positive charges, the milliequivalent concentration of Ca^{2+} is 4 mEq/L (2 mmol/L × 2 positive charges per Ca molecule). Similarly, the milliequivalent concentration of Cl^- is also 4 mEq/L (the 4 total Cl^- × 1 negative charge per Cl^-). Conversely, it is a simple matter to divide the concentration in mEq/L by the charge per ion to get the millimolar concentration.

Using mOsm/L. To determine the osmolarity of a solution, multiply the millimolar concentration by the number of particles into which the substance dissolves. The 2 mmol/L $CaCl_2$ solution described dissociates into three particles (i.e., $Ca^{2+} + Cl^- + Cl^-$). Thus, for every mmol/L, there are three particles. Because there are 2 mmol/L, the milliosmolar concentration is 6 mOsm/L (2 mmol/L × 3 particles/mmol).

In summary, a 22.2 mg/dL $CaCl_2$ solution contains 2 mmol/L $CaCl_2$, 4 mEq/L of Ca^{2+} and 4 mEq/L of Cl^-, and has a concentration of 6 mOsm/L.

Electrochemical Gradient

Molecules tend to diffuse from an area of high molecular concentration to one of lower concentration. They are said to diffuse "down" their chemical concentration gradient. Charged molecules also move down their electrical gradients (Fig. 1-6).

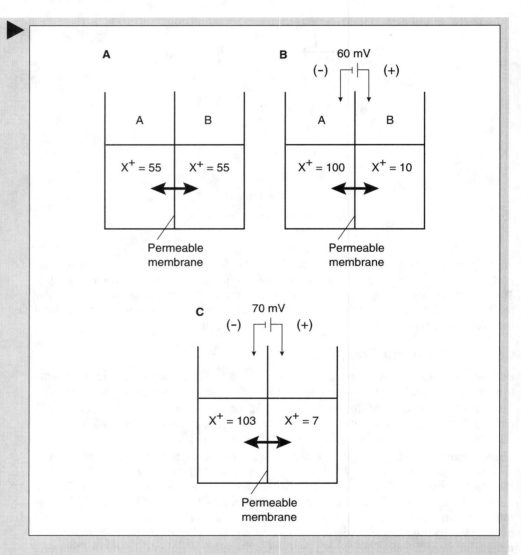

FIGURE 1-6

Electrochemical Equilibrium is the Balance between Concentration and Electrical Differences. (A) There are two compartments of equal size separated by a membrane permeable to X^+. At equilibrium, the concentration of X^+ on both sides of the membrane is the same because of diffusion, and no further net movement of X^+ occurs. (B) Application of a 60 mV potential across the membrane results in a net movement of X^+. Charged molecules also move down their electrical gradient as well as their chemical gradient. The membrane has an electrical potential across it, and compartment A is negative relative to compartment B. The source of the potential difference is irrelevant; it could be caused by a battery. The negative potential in compartment A tends to attract X^+ because of the positive charge, and the positive potential in compartment B tends to repel X^+. Therefore, the concentration of X^+ in compartment A increases, and the concentration of X^+ in compartment B decreases. Thus, there is a net electrochemical gradient acting on X^+. At equilibrium, the electrical gradient tending to move X^+ from compartment B to compartment A is balanced by the chemical gradient tending to move X^+ from compartment A to compartment B, so there is no net movement of X^+. The ions are in electrochemical equilibrium, which is the balance between the chemical concentration difference and the electrical potential difference acting on charged molecules. (C) If, however, the potential difference across the barrier increases further (to 70 mV), the increased negative charge in compartment A would again tend to promote the movement of the positive X^+ from compartment B to compartment A, and the concentration difference would increase until the electrochemical gradient again reached equilibrium.

There are many instances in the kidney in which the chemical and the electrical gradients oppose each other, and there are many instances in which they reinforce each other and act in the same direction. As one example, many cations are reabsorbed against their chemical concentration gradient in the thick ascending limb of Henle because the basolateral side is negative relative to the lumen. The positive cations are attracted to the relative negative charge outside and repelled by the positive charge inside the limb. The cations move between the cells down their electrical gradient and are reabsorbed. The equilibrium conditions shown in Fig. 1-6 can be mathematically derived using biophysical principles and the Nernst equation. Exploration of these principles is beyond the scope of this book, but a further explanation can be found in any neurophysiology text. However, they are unnecessary for the understanding of renal physiology, as long as one grasps the concepts.

BODY FLUID COMPARTMENTS

Composition

Before delving into the mechanisms of renal regulation, it is also necessary to have a grasp of some of the many normal constituents of the body fluid volumes that the kidney regulates; in particular, those of the extracellular volume. A partial listing of the ECF components and their normal values is given in Table 1-3. These values have been obtained from venous plasma samples, with the assumption that the plasma composition of electrolytes is nearly identical to the rest of the extracellular space. Although this is a simple assumption, it is sometimes not appreciated. The range of values may vary, however, depending on the particular laboratory used for analysis.

◀ **TABLE 1-3**
Typical Plasma Values

Substance	Range of Values	Average Values
Sodium	135–145 mEq/L	140
Chloride	95–107 mEq/L	100
Bicarbonate	23–29 mEq/L	24
Osmolarity	275–295 mOsm/L	280
Potassium	3.8–5.1 mEq/L	4
Calcium	2.24–2.46 mEq/L	2.4
Phosphorus	2.7–4.5 mg/dL	4
pH	7.35–7.45	7.4
Creatinine	0.7–1.3 mg%	1
Blood urea nitrogen	7–18 mg%	15
Anion gap ($Na^+-Cl^--HCO_3^-$)	10–16 mEq/L	13

Several of these values need elaboration. Na^+ is the major cation in the ECF. As such, Na^+ and the accompanying Cl^- and HCO_3^- anions are primarily responsible for the extracellular osmolarity. Gains or losses of water from the body that alter extracellular osmolarity almost always result in changes in extracellular Na^+ concentration. However, there are a few exceptions, such as elevated glucose in patients with uncontrolled diabetes.

In most cases, plasma Na^+ concentration is an indication of extracellular osmolarity.

Also, the total concentration of the major cation (Na^+) does not equal the total concentration of the major anions (Cl^- + HCO_3^-). The so called *anion gap* is given in Table 1-3. This does not mean that the other anions are not there, but that they are simply not measured in routine chemical analysis. As discussed in a later chapter, a larger-than-normal concentration of unmeasured anions (anion gap) is a technique used in a clinical setting to determine the cause of many acid–base disturbances.

Both creatinine and BUN are by-products of metabolism. They increase as renal function decreases, and as will be discussed later, they also can be used to evaluate renal function. A disproportionate increase in BUN relative to creatinine is used many times to differentiate between severe plasma volume contraction and developing renal failure. Under normal conditions, these by-products are removed from the body by glomerular filtration.

Although it is relatively easy to assess the components of the ECF from a simple blood sample, the measurement of the intracellular components is much more problematic. How does one get a representative sample of K^+ from the cell? It is very difficult, and

Intracellular concentrations are difficult to measure.

most values given for concentrations inside the cells are educated guesses or estimated from analysis of whole tissue samples. The educated guesses are, however, very good guesses. K^+ concentration inside the cells is known to be higher than K^+ outside the cells because of the Na^+-K^+-ATPase that actively pumps K^+ into the cells and pumps Na^+ out of the cells. Because of the Na^+-K^+-ATPase, the Na^+ concentration inside the cells is low, and almost all Na^+ in the body is in the ECF. Cytosolic Ca^{2+} inside the cells is known to be 10,000 times lower than Ca^{2+} outside the cells because the intracellular Ca^{2+} is sequestered mainly in the endoplasmic reticulum and also is extruded from the cell by Na^+-Ca^{2+} exchange and Ca^{2+}-ATPase. In addition, the extracellular Cl^- concentration is known to be much higher than the intracellular concentration because the electrochemical gradient for Cl^- moves Cl^- into the ECF. Finally, the pH inside the cell is known to be lower than pH outside the cells because intracellular metabolism generates H^+ ions.

Volume

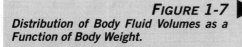

*The **60-40-20 rule** is used as a rough approximation of body fluid volumes based on weight. Approximately 60% of the body weight is water; 40% is intracellular, and 20% is extracellular.*

In its simplest concept, water in the body can exist only in two places. It can be either inside the cells as intracellular volume or outside the cells as extracellular volume. This relationship is shown as a box diagram in Fig. 1-7. For practical purposes, distribution of body water follows an approximate 60-40-20 rule. For a normal individual, approximately 60% of body weight is water; approximately 40% is intracellular, and 20% is extracellular. Because 1 L of water weighs 1 kg, it follows that 60% of a 70-kg person results in 42 kg (or 42 L) of total body water. If 40% of the body is intracellular water, then the intracellular volume is approximately 28 L, and the extracellular volume is approximately 14 L. Also, the distribution of water between the two compartments is roughly two-thirds intracellular and one-third extracellular. This rule is very useful, applies to different-sized subjects, and is rather consistent among different species. A 2-kg rabbit would have a total body water of approximately 1.2 L, which is approximately 60% of body weight. Obviously, very young infants, who are mostly water, will have a higher percentage of their body weight as water, and obese patients will have a lower percentage because adipose tissue has very little water content. As a general rule, normal men have a slightly higher percentage of their body weight as water than normal women. Nevertheless, the compartmentalization between intracellular fluid (ICF) and ECF does not change appreciably. Also illustrated in Fig. 1-7 is the blood volume, which represents approximately 8% of body weight. A portion of the volume in the cardiovascular system is extracellular and is represented by the plasma volume, whereas the other portion of the

FIGURE 1-7 ▶
Distribution of Body Fluid Volumes as a Function of Body Weight.

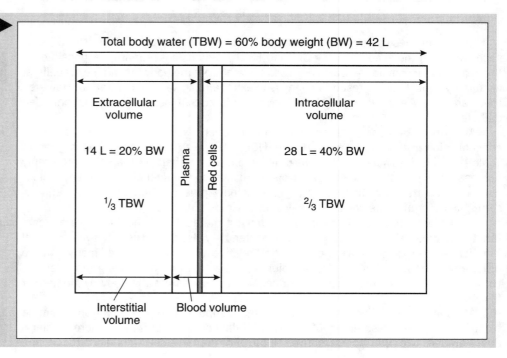

volume is inside the RBCs and thus, intracellular. The relative portion of the blood volume that is RBCs is easily determined from the hematocrit. The portion of the extracellular volume that is not plasma is the interstitial volume.

Measurement

Body fluid volumes are determined by a technique called *indicator dilution* (Fig. 1-8A), which depends on the assumption of conservation of mass. Fig. 1-8B shows a helpful relationship between concentration, amount, and volume. If the volume of fluid in the bottle shown in Fig. 1-8A needs to be known but cannot be emptied, a known amount of a substance that is not lost from the bottle could be added and allowed to equilibrate with the fluid. The final concentration can then be measured, and the volume can be calculated. In the example shown in Fig. 1-8A, 2 mEq of Na^+ are added, and the final concentration is determined to be 0.5 mEq/L. The volume can be calculated as follows: volume = amount/concentration = 2mEq/0.5 mEq/L = 4L.

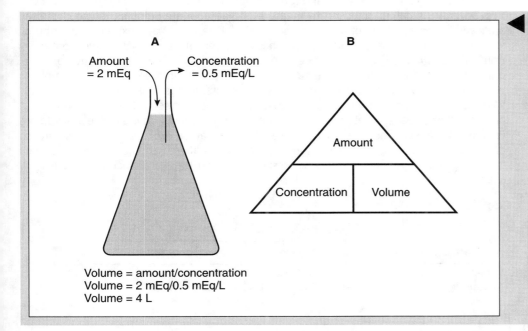

Volume = amount/concentration
Volume = 2 mEq/0.5 mEq/L
Volume = 4 L

◄ **FIGURE 1-8**
(A) Example of indicator dilution technique for measuring volume. (B) Triangle relating amount, concentration, and volume. Cover up concentration, and you have amount divided by volume. Cover up amount, and you have concentration times volume.

With some modifications to this indicator dilution method, the same approach is used to measure the body fluid volumes. A known amount of an indicator is injected into a vein, allowed sufficient time to equilibrate, and a representative plasma sample is obtained after equilibration. The concentration is measured, and it is then a simple matter to calculate the volume in which the indicator was diluted. Two caveats must be considered when applying this technique to living subjects. First, the only reasonable access to obtain a representative sample of the final concentration of the indicator is from a blood sample. If the indicator is taken up by the cells, then the dilution will be determined by the intracellular volume. Since a representative sample cannot be taken from the cells, it follows that intracellular volume cannot be directly measured. Second, in the example in Fig. 1-8A, Na^+ was assumed to be not lost (i.e., conservation of mass). However, Na^+ is lost from the body by continued renal excretion. Most indicators used to measure body fluid volumes are lost through the kidneys, and the loss sustained during equilibration must be determined or estimated.

Measurement of the extracellular volume is rather straightforward. A small amount of radioactive Na^+ is injected into the vein, allowed sufficient time to equilibrate, and a plasma concentration is subsequently obtained. A urine sample can be collected to estimate the amount of radioactive Na^+ lost through the kidneys. The amount of radioactive Na^+ remaining after equilibrium is determined by subtracting the urine loss from the initial amount injected. The volume is determined by dividing the amount remaining in

Indicator Dilution Technique. If a known amount of an appropriate indicator is injected into the body and allowed to equilibrate, the volume in which the indicator is diluted can be determined by measuring the final concentration after equilibrium and dividing it into the amount injected.

the body by the final concentration. This can be stated mathematically by the following relationship:

$$Volume = (amount\ in - amount\ lost) / final\ concentration$$

Because Na+ is confined to the extracellular space, radioactive Na+ can be used to estimate the extracellular volume. It is common practice in many cases to estimate the urine loss or ignore it altogether if the plasma sample is taken soon after the injection.

Similar methods are used to measure plasma volume and total body water. For plasma volume, labeled albumin is injected into the vein, and a plasma sample is obtained for measurement of labeled albumin. Because albumin is primarily confined to the cardiovascular volume, the plasma volume can be determined. Total body water can be measured by tritiated water using the same methodology as measurement of extracellular volume. However, quantitation of water loss from the body resulting from respiration, perspiration, GI secretions, and renal excretion is difficult at best.

Several indicators are used to measure the appropriate volumes; some of these are given in Table 1-4. All of the substances listed in Table 1-4 approximately distribute in the appropriate spaces indicated, and sometimes the term "volume of distribution" is used when discussing volumes. For instance, the volume of distribution of Na+ implies extracellular volume, whereas the volume of distribution of albumin implies plasma volume. A similar extra terminology also exists; that is, the concept of "space." When using Na+ as an indicator, it must be recognized that some Na+ enters the cell, and the Na+ "space" that is measured would be an overestimation of extracellular volume. Conversely, inulin is a large molecule that may be excluded from some areas of the extracellular volume. The inulin "space" is smaller than the Na+ space. The true extracellular volume is surely somewhere between the Na+ space and the inulin space.

> *Na+ "space" is the volume in which the Na+ in the body is distributed.*

TABLE 1-4 ▶
Substances Used to Measure Volumes

Extracellular Volume	Plasma Volume	Total Body Water
Radiolabeled sodium	Iodinated albumin	Tritiated water
Sucrose	T-1824 (Evans blue)	Heavy water
Mannitol		Antipyrine
Inulin		

Because the plasma volume and the ECF volume are rather easy to measure, they can be used to calculate two additional volumes—the blood volume and the interstitial volume. *Blood volume* is defined as plasma volume/(1 − hematocrit). *Interstitial fluid volume* is the difference between ECF volume and plasma volume. ICF volume is also the difference between total body water and the ECF volume.

Osmotic Shifts

Under normal conditions, the body fluid volumes remain very constant. However, there are times when renal function is compromised, input is altered, or plasma osmolarity is changed by metabolic disturbances such as diabetes. In these circumstances, changes in body fluid composition can have profound effects on body fluid volumes. Cells in the body change volume in response to their osmotic environment. The effect of changing the external osmolarity on RBC volume is shown in Fig. 1-9. Placing the isotonic cell in a hypotonic solution results in movement of water from outside the cell into the cell, and the cell swells until the osmolarity of the external solution and the internal solution are equal (A → B). Placing a similar cell into a hypertonic solution results in movement of water from inside the cell, and the cell shrinks until the osmolarity of the external solution and the internal solution are equal (C → D).

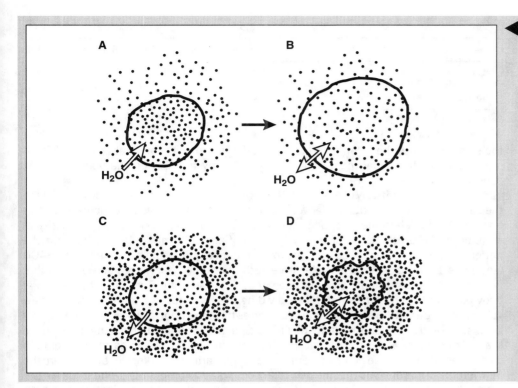

FIGURE 1-9
Effect of Placing a Cell in a Nonisotonic Solution. *A cell in a hypotonic NaCl solution swells (A → B). A cell in a hypertonic NaCl solution shrinks (C → D). Water moves until the osmolarities inside and outside the cell are equal.*

Body Fluid Volume Shifts

Just as a single RBC changes volume in response to an osmotic challenge, so do all the cells in the body. Correction of volume disorders, which can occur during severe dehydration, vomiting, diarrhea, or diabetes insipidus, requires a knowledge of the volume shifts that may be encountered. There are three points that must be considered to work through the volume shifts.

*In **equilibrium conditions**, the osmolarity of the ECF volume and the ICF volume are equal.*

1. It must be understood where the water and solute are distributed. For example, an infusion of a concentrated solution of K^+ results in most of the K^+ being taken up by the cells because of the Na^+-K^+-ATPase in the cell membrane. Infused Na^+ remains outside the cells because of the same mechanism, whereas water is distributed between both the intracellular and the extracellular volume. Solutions containing metabolizable solutes, such as glucose, or membrane permeable solutes, such as urea, eventually distribute similarly to water.

2. The second consideration concerns the whole body osmotic equilibrium. Because of the tremendous effect of osmotic concentration differences to move water, the osmolarity in the ECF comes to equilibrium with the osmolarity of the ICF. The movement of water is very rapid, and equilibration occurs within a matter of minutes. Thus, the osmolarity of the total body water comes to equilibrium very quickly.

3. Finally, the individual volumes can be determined from a knowledge of the whole body fluid osmolarity at equilibrium and the amount of solute in each compartment. Some examples of body volume fluid shifts are given below.

Increased Water Intake. A 50-kg student has excessive thirst (polydipsia). After leaving an examination, his body fluid volumes are normal, but he stops at a water fountain and drinks 2 L of water. What are his normal volumes and osmolarity before drinking the water and what are they after the water is absorbed?

Because his body fluid volumes are normal, his plasma osmolarity is approximately 280 mOsm/L. This is also the osmolarity of the extracellular and intracellular volume and, by inference, his total body water. The 60-40-20 rule then can be applied to estimate his volumes. Because he weighs 50 kg, his total body water is approximately 60% of 50 kg, or 30 L. His intracellular volume is approximately 40% of his body weight (20 L), whereas his extracellular volume is approximately 10 L. This relationship between the variables is given in Table 1-5. Note that the osmolarity in all compartments is

TABLE 1-5 ▶
Body Fluid Volume and Composition

	Volume (L)	Concentration (mOsm/L)	Amount (mOsm)
Extracellular	10	280	2800
Intracellular	20	280	5600
Total body water	30	280	8400

the same. Because the volume and concentration are known, the total amount of milliosmoles in each compartment can be calculated by multiplying the volume by the concentration (see Fig. 1-8B).

Addition of water to the body decreases osmolarity and increases both the extracellular and intracellular volume.

It should be intuitively obvious that the ingested water distributes inside and outside the cells, and both the extracellular volume and the intracellular volume increase. But by how much? To determine this, one must keep track of whole body fluid osmolarity at equilibrium. The osmolarity of the body was initially 280 mOsm/L and, because the patient's body contained 30 L water, the total amount of milliosmoles in the body is 8400 (see Table 1-5). No osmotic particles were added with the 2 L of ingested water, so that now the 8400 mOsm solute are contained in 32 L. As shown in Table 1-6, the new total body osmolarity can be determined by dividing the total number of mOsm by the new volume, giving a value of 263 mOsm/L. As soon as the absorption of water from the GI tract begins, the extracellular osmolarity begins to decrease, and the higher osmolarity inside the cells promotes water movement into the cells until the two compartments come to osmotic equilibrium. The new osmolarity of both compartments is known, but what are the new volumes? It is obvious that the new total body water volume is 32 L, and it is a simple matter to calculate the individual volumes. The total number of milliosmoles in both compartments is known, as is the new osmolarity. Exactly like the indicator dilution technique discussed previously, the volume can be calculated by dividing the amount by the concentration. The new extracellular volume, therefore, is 10.6 L. Because the total body water is 32 L, and 10.6 L are extracellular, then the rest must be in the intracellular space. This difference is 21.4 L. These new relationships are summarized in Table 1-6.

TABLE 1-6 ▶
New Volume and Composition after Ingestion of 2 L of Water

	Volume (L)	Concentration (mOsm/L)	Amount (mOsm)
Extracellular	10.6	263	2800
Intracellular	21.4	263	5600
Total body water	32.0	263	8400

In a healthy individual, the kidney excretes the excess water and returns the volumes and composition to normal in a relatively short period of time. However, it should be recognized that in a patient with renal impairment, excess water may not be excreted efficiently, resulting in long-term changes in osmolarity and volume of both the extracellular and intracellular compartments.

Hypertonic NaCl Infusion. A 60-kg patient is admitted to the hospital for routine outpatient surgery. A blood sample reveals that he has a normal plasma osmolarity of 280 mOsm/L. He is supposed to be infused with 1 L of isotonic saline for preoperative hydration. Instead, a mistake is made, and he is given 2 L of a 500 mmol/L NaCl solution used to treat hyponatremia.

• What are the body fluid volumes and osmolarities before and after the infusion?

The 60-40-20 rule can be used to estimate the volumes, and the osmolarity is given. These values are given in Table 1-7. Again, it is necessary to understand where the infused substance goes. In this case, both solute and water are added to the body. Because the infusion is NaCl, the particles are confined almost exclusively to the extracellular volume. The NaCl solution has a concentration of 500 mmol/L of NaCl. NaCl exists in solution as Na^+ and Cl^-. Thus, for every millimole of NaCl in solution there are

TABLE 1-7
Body Fluid Volume and Composition

	Volume (L)	Concentration (mOsm/L)	Amount (mOsm)
Extracellular	12	280	3360
Intracellular	24	280	6720
Total body water	36	280	10,080

two particles. Therefore, each liter, which has a 500 mmol/L concentration of NaCl, has an osmotic concentration of 1000 mOsm/L. Because 2 L were infused, there was a total of 2000 mOsm added to the total body, but it is confined primarily to the extracellular volume. The first step in determining the new volumes and osmolarity is to determine the new whole body osmotic equilibrium value, which is shown in Table 1-8.

TABLE 1-8
New Volume and Composition after Infusion of 2 L of 500 mmol/L NaCl

	Volume (L)	Concentration (mOsm/L)	Amount (mOsm)
Total body water	36	280	10,080
Added	2	1000	2000
Equilibrium	38	318	12,080

Adding the 2 L increased the total body water from 36 to 38 L, and adding the 2000 mOsm increased the total body milliosmoles from 10,080 to 12,080. As in the water ingestion circumstance given above, the osmotic concentration at equilibrium is determined by dividing the total milliosmoles by the new volume to give a new osmotic concentration of 318 mOsm/L. Similar logic can be used to determine the new extracellular volume as shown in Table 1-9.

TABLE 1-9
New Extracellular Volume after Addition of 2 L of Hypertonic Saline

	Volume (L)	Concentration (mOsm/L)	Amount (mOsm)
Extracellular	12	280	3360
Added	2	1000	2000
Equilibrium	16.9	318	5360

Because all the osmotic particles were added to the extracellular volume, the total number of milliosmoles in the extracellular volume increased by 2000 mOsm. The increased extracellular osmolarity resulted in osmotic movement of water from the intracellular volume to the extracellular volume until osmotic equilibrium was reached. Dividing the total extracellular milliosmoles by the new concentration yields the new volume of 16.9 L. The difference between the new total body water (38 L) and the new extracellular volume (16.9 L) gives the new intracellular volume of 21.1 L.

Infusion of the hyperosmotic solution increased the extracellular volume but also increased the extracellular osmolarity. Although 2 L volume was infused, the hypertonic solution actually dehydrated the cells, and the extracellular volume further increased at the expense of the intracellular volume.

Although this example used an extreme perturbation, it emphasized the point that the osmolarity of any solution should be considered when infused into the body because of the osmotic shifts that may occur. A knowledge of osmotic shifts also may be useful in a clinical setting. In a patient with acute head trauma and cerebral edema, it is possible to decrease the intracranial pressure and volume by infusion of a concentrated solution of mannitol. Mannitol is an inert sugar that is not metabolized by the body and, thus, remains outside the cells. The increased extracellular osmolarity results in movement of water out of the neurons, which decreases the intracellular edema. Because the mannitol is rapidly excreted by the kidney, the effect may be short-term. However, it may be

Addition of a hypertonic NaCl solution to the body increases osmolarity and increases the extracellular volume at the expense of the intracellular volume.

lifesaving until other measures can be taken. Finally, there are some pathologic conditions in which fluid shifts occur. Perhaps the most common is the acute increase in extracellular glucose in patients with uncontrolled diabetes mellitus. The increased extracellular glucose results in increased extracellular osmolarity, a movement of water out of the cells, and intracellular dehydration.

Severe Sweating. A football player undergoes a strenuous pre-season workout on a hot August afternoon, and he sweats profusely. During the final wind sprints, he collapses and is taken to the emergency department. On admission, he is still sweating but his skin is pale. His plasma osmolarity is 310 mOsm/L, his plasma Na+ concentration is 146 mEq/L, and he weighs 100 kg. The diagnosis is dehydration due to excessive sweating.

In many ways, this example is a reverse of the two situations above. What must be determined is the volume and composition of the fluids that must be administered to correct the volume deficit rather than determine the volume shifts that occur after fluid administration. The first consideration is how much water must be given to correct the increased osmolarity that resulted from the lost fluid; the second consideration is the resulting plasma Na+ concentration. Sweat is a hypotonic fluid that is basically derived from the ECF, and its major function is to maintain thermal homeostasis by evaporative cooling. Because it is hypotonic, excessive sweating leads to concentration of the body fluids. As the extracellular osmolarity increases, water is removed from the cells until whole body osmotic equilibrium occurs. Even a person who is heat acclimated may produce a very dilute fluid, but sweat is not pure water. Therefore, the football player has undoubtedly also lost some Na+.

> Loss of water from the body increases osmolarity and decreases both extracellular and intracellular volume.

Consider the correction of the water deficit first. How much water is necessary to return the plasma osmolarity to a normal 280 mOsm/L? Is it 1 L or 20 L or somewhere in between? Because the patient has lost fluid, the total body water is probably less than 60% of his body weight. However, for this example, assume that the 100-kg subject begins with a total body water of 60 L. The total number of milliosmoles is then 60 L × 310 mOsm/L for a total of 18,600 mOsm. In the triangle in Fig. 1-8B, it can be seen that the total volume necessary to achieve a concentration of 280 mOsm/L can be calculated by dividing the amount by the concentration. Thus, 18,600 mOsm/280 mOsm/L = 66 L. Therefore, the patient needs to have at least an additional 6 L of water to return the plasma osmolarity to near normal.

Assuming the patient has 20% of his body weight as ECF, then the extracellular volume is 20 L and contains 146 mEq/L of Na+. The total Na+ in the extracellular volume is 2920 mEq. The volume required to achieve normal osmolarity is the addition of 6 L of water, as determined above. As illustrated in Fig. 1-7, approximately one-third of this water is distributed in the extracellular volume. After the addition of the water, the extracellular volume is increased to 22 L. What is the resulting Na+ concentration? It is the total amount of Na+ (2920 mEq) divided by the new volume (22 L). The result is an unacceptable Na+ concentration of 133 mEq/L. Therefore, Na+ also must be added, but how much? If the desired Na+ concentration is a normal plasma Na+ concentration of approximately 140 mEq/L, then 7 mEq must be added for each liter of ECF. Because there are approximately 22 L of ECF, the patient needs a total of 154 mEq of Na+.

Although the example is rife with assumptions, they are reasonable assumptions. Surely, the total body water is less than 60% of the body weight and may be around 55%, but a 5% error is acceptable and gives a starting point for therapy. The infused Na+ also results in increased extracellular volume because of the osmotic effect of the extracellular Na+. In practice, the fluids should be given slowly, the outcome should be closely monitored, and corrections should be made as necessary.

A widely held assumption, particularly among those with a poor knowledge of body fluid volumes, is that excessive sweating should be followed with salt tablets. It is easy to see how this thought process was derived. As water evaporates, the electrolytes are left on the skin, and perspiration tastes salty. However, salt tablets are exactly the wrong treatment because the body is losing hypotonic fluid. Because salt tablets increase extracellular Na+ concentration and osmolarity, they result in further increased intracellular dehydration and increased total body osmolarity. Increased water intake and a little salt with the following meal is much more appropriate.

Graphic Analysis of Volume Shifts. Changes in body fluid volumes and composition often are represented in diagrammatic form, and these diagrams are used to test the understanding of what has occurred. Fig. 1-10 illustrates the changes that occur following water ingestion, hypertonic NaCl infusion, dehydration, and hypotonic NaCl infusion. Using the box in Fig. 1-7 to represent body fluid volumes, it becomes a simple matter to put units on the box. The volume of each compartment is represented by the x-axis, and osmolarity is represented by the y-axis. The solid box represents the control conditions, whereas the dotted lines represent the equilibrium conditions after the perturbations. Total solute in each compartment is simply the product of the osmotic concentration multiplied by the compartment volume. Following water ingestion, the volume of both the extracellular and intracellular compartment increases, and the whole body osmolarity decreases (see Fig. 1-10A). As seen in Fig. 1-10B, addition of a hypertonic solution, which remains in the extracellular volume, results in an increase in extracellular volume at the expense of a decrease in the intracellular volume, whereas whole body osmolarity increases. Dehydration from sweating or an inability to ingest water results in a decrease in both extracellular and intracellular volume and an increase in whole body osmolarity (see Fig. 1-10C). Although a specific example for addition of hypotonic NaCl was not given in the examples above, it should be appreciated that the effect is qualitatively similar to water. An increase in both extracellular

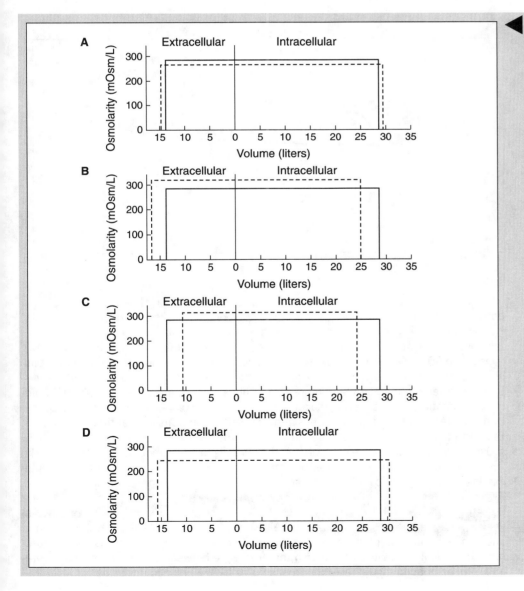

◀ ***FIGURE 1-10***
Graphic Representation of the Relationships between Body Fluid Volumes and Osmolarity. Solid lines *represent the control conditions. The* dotted lines *represent the equilibrium conditions following (A) addition of water, (B) addition of a hypertonic NaCl solution, (C) loss of pure water, and (D) addition of hypotonic NaCl solution.*

and intracellular volume occurs along with a decrease in total body osmolarity, as depicted in Fig. 1-10D. It should also be appreciated that an iso-osmotic solution of NaCl increases the extracellular volume and maintains both the intracellular volume and the whole body osmolarity constant.

Colloid Osmotic Pressure versus Osmolarity. One of the most common mistakes made when considering osmotic shifts is to confuse the osmotic pressure resulting from small solutes with the osmotic pressure resulting from proteins. The movement of fluid into and out of cells is governed by the solute concentration differences across cell membranes and was illustrated in Fig. 1-9. The movement of fluid across capillaries is due to the osmotic pressure from protein concentration differences and hydrostatic pressure differences across the capillary (Fig. 1-11). The difference in protein concentration across the capillary exerts an osmotic pressure called the colloid osmotic or the oncotic pressure and is often abbreviated as pi (π). Because the capillary is relatively impermeable to the proteins, they generate an osmotic pressure to cause water to move from a region with low colloid osmotic pressure, such as the interstitium, to high colloid osmotic pressure, such as the plasma. In systemic capillaries the colloid osmotic pressure is nearly balanced by the hydrostatic pressures surrounding the capillaries, and there is very little net water movement across the capillary wall. It is the balance of these pressures that is responsible for the maintenance of plasma volume.

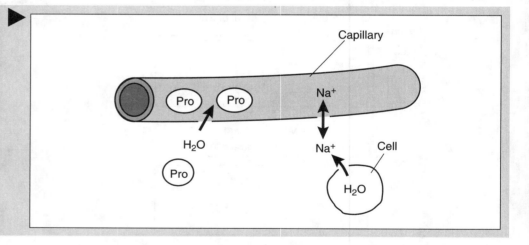

FIGURE 1-11 ▶

Relationship between the Colloid Osmotic Pressure Resulting from Protein (Pro) Concentration on Fluid Movement Across a Capillary Wall and Osmotic Pressure Resulting from Small Solutes Such as Na+ on Fluid Movements across Cell Membranes. *Protein concentration differences tend to move fluid across the capillary. The Na+ is free to diffuse and exerts no osmotic pressure at the capillary. At the cell, excess Na+ can exert an osmotic pressure, causing water to move out of the cell.*

Because the capillary is permeable to small solutes, changing the plasma osmolarity does not affect water movement across the capillary because the small solutes such as Na+ are free to diffuse or be carried across the capillary by bulk fluid flow. In contrast, an increase in plasma osmolarity (and by inference extracellular osmolarity) from 280 mOsm/L to 300 mOsm/L exerts a very large osmotic pressure to move fluid out of the cells and decrease intracellular volume. However, the increased plasma osmolarity has virtually no effect on capillary fluid movement. Conversely, an increase in interstitial fluid colloid osmotic pressure, as might occur during lymphatic blockade, has a large effect on transcapillary fluid movement but has almost no effect on transcellular fluid movement. Even in plasma, the osmotic concentration of protein is low and on the order of 1.5 mOsm/L, which is negligible compared to the normal plasma osmolarity of approximately 280 mOsm/L. The proteins in the plasma are large molecules, and a large molecule exerts the same osmotic pressure as a small molecule across an impermeable membrane. Because the hydrostatic pressures surrounding the capillary are small, the small colloid osmotic pressure resulting from the proteins is important in the regulation of plasma volume, although it is the total osmolarity that alters intracellular volume. The volume and composition of fluid moved across the glomerular capillary are discussed in detail later, but it is important to distinguish the difference between colloid osmotic pressure and total osmotic pressure resulting from solutes before proceeding further.

RESOLUTION OF CLINICAL CASES

Case 1

In any clinical condition, a physical examination is extremely valuable and usually points the way to future considerations. In Case 1 the history and physical signs pointed to severe dehydration of some duration. The patient had a history of stroke and a broken hip, which made ambulation difficult. She may have had another stroke, which made it impossible for her to walk and ingest water. In addition, she may have been in this condition for several days because her friends had not seen her for that long. The blood pressure was low and may be indicative of plasma volume contraction. The heart rate was very elevated, most probably as a result of increased sympathetic nervous system output in response to the decreased plasma volume and blood pressure. Finally, she gave the impression of being dry or dehydrated because of the poor skin elasticity and very dry mouth.

Routine chemical analysis of venous plasma usually results in a panel of the seven determined values given in the case. There are five striking laboratory findings. The BUN, creatinine, Na^+, and Cl^- levels were remarkably elevated, and there was no urine output. As discussed earlier in the chapter, BUN and creatinine are both metabolic by-products that are removed from the body by filtration in a healthy kidney. The BUN was approximately ten times normal, and the creatinine level was approximately four times normal. Those observations coupled with the absence of urine output almost surely point to acute renal failure as a result of severe volume depletion and sympathetic nervous system constriction of the kidney. Most likely the kidneys were functional, but they were severely compromised by the low renal blood flow resulting from the constriction.

The most likely life-threatening situation is a very elevated plasma osmolarity. Although a plasma osmolarity is not given, the high Na^+ concentration suggests that it was increased. Na^+ and its anions are by far the largest determinants of extracellular osmolarity. Many clinical laboratories do not routinely perform a measurement of plasma osmolarity. In fact, many small medical practices do not have the facilities to measure any osmolarity at all. Urine osmolarity can be estimated by specific gravity of the urine measured with a floating hydrometer. The higher the specific gravity, the more concentrated the urine. Moreover, plasma osmolarity can be estimated from the data given. The major particles that determine measured osmolarity are the Na^+ and the K^+ plus their anions and the osmotic concentration of the urea and glucose. To account for the anions, the Na^+ and K^+ must be multiplied by 2. The molecular weight of the nitrogen derived from the BUN is 28 mg/mmol, and the molecular weight of glucose is 180 mg/mmol. Because the values from this clinical laboratory were reported in mg/100 mL for both BUN and glucose, the concentration of BUN must be divided by 2.8, and glucose must be divided by 18 to get the units of mOsm/L. The final calculation for plasma osmolarity (P_{Osm}) becomes:

$$P_{Osm} = 2 \times (Na^+ + K^+) + BUN/2.8 + glucose/18$$

$$P_{Osm} = 2 \times (170 + 4.1) + 120/2.8 + 90/18 = 396 \text{ mOsm/L}$$

There has been a severe loss of water and a resulting increase in extracellular osmolarity in this patient. The marked increase in extracellular osmolarity resulting from the water loss removed water from the cells and resulted in marked intracellular dehydration. The inability to ingest water in the face of continued water loss also resulted in extracellular dehydration. The disorientation, unconsciousness, and inability to answer questions was almost certainly due to the neural dehydration. The most obvious treatment is to replace the water the patient was unable to obtain.

The calculation of the osmolarity used above may be considered cumbersome. However, in the absence of a measured plasma osmolarity, it can be very useful in the diagnosis and treatment of osmolar disturbances. As an initial approach, the plasma Na^+ concentration alone can be used as an estimation of plasma osmolarity. Although the glucose in this patient was relatively unimportant in the determination of plasma osmolarity, it becomes very important in situations, such as diabetes, when plasma glucose increases. This case also emphasizes the importance of intake in the everyday regulation of water balance. Everyone undergoes water loss, whether by respiration, perspiration, or through the kidneys. Even in the relatively short term, total water deprivation can have serious consequences on the kidneys' ability to regulate the volume and composition of the body fluids because, in the absence of input, the kidney can only minimize losses.

Case 2

Because of worsening clinical problems, the patient was treated by dialysis. Whether treated by hemodialysis or peritoneal dialysis, most patients lead reasonably normal and productive lives. It should be appreciated by now that dialysis treatment requires strict adherence to the treatment regimen to be fully successful. The most obvious solution is a successful kidney transplant.

REVIEW QUESTIONS

Directions: For each of the following questions, choose the **one best** answer.

1. Infusion of a hypertonic NaCl solution decreases which one of the following body fluid volumes?

    (A) Interstitial volume

    (B) Extracellular volume

    (C) Intracellular volume

    (D) Total body water

2. A 2 mmol/L solution of $CaCl_2$ has a concentration of

    (A) 4 mEq/L of Ca^{2+}, 6 mOsm/L

    (B) 4 mg%, 2 mEq/L Ca^{2+}

    (C) 4 mOsm/L, 6 mEq/L Ca^{2+}

    (D) 2 mEq/L of Cl^-, 6 mOsm/L

3. A patient with severe renal failure and protein loss in the urine might be expected to have

    (A) increased hematocrit

    (B) increased plasma creatinine concentration

    (C) decreased plasma K^+ concentration

    (D) increased plasma volume

4. A well-conditioned 80-kg athlete pitched a baseball game and subsequently lost 3 kg. If the plasma osmolarity was 300 mOsm/L when he started the game, what was the approximate plasma osmolarity when he finished the game if the loss consisted of pure water?

    (A) 369 mOsm/L

    (B) 331 mOsm/L

    (C) 320 mOsm/L

    (D) 312 mOsm/L

5. A pediatric patient who weighs 10 kg is injected with 3 g of drug Z. One hour later, 1 g of the drug is found in the urine. At this time, the plasma concentration is 1 mg/mL. It would appear that drug Z is distributed in the

    (A) plasma volume

    (B) extracellular volume

    (C) intracellular volume

    (D) total body water

6. Use the graphic analysis below to answer this question. If the *solid lines* represent the normal condition, which one of the following actions is represented by the dashed lines?

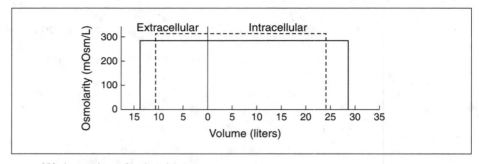

(A) Ingestion of salt tablets

(B) Ingestion of excess water

(C) Severe sweating

(D) Drinking a sports beverage to replace electrolyte loss

7. An increase in the negative electrical potential in compartment A in the figure below from −70 mV to −80 mV causes the movement of the positive molecule X^+ across the membrane separating the compartments. Therefore, which one of the following scenarios will occur?

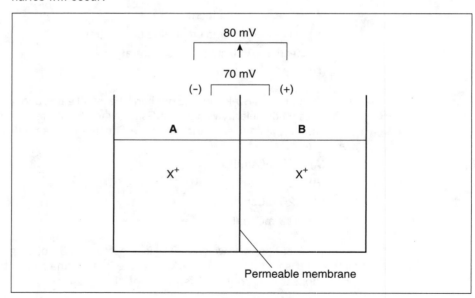

(A) The concentration of X^+ in compartment A will decrease.

(B) The concentration difference of X^+ between the compartments will decrease.

(C) The concentration of X^+ in compartment B will decrease.

(D) The potential difference will increase.

8. Beaker A contains a 100 mOsm/L solution. Beaker B contains a 280 mOsm/L solution. Beaker C contains a 1200 mOsm/L solution. Which one of the following statements is true?

(A) Beaker B is isotonic and also hypo-osmotic compared to beaker A.

(B) Beaker C is hypotonic and also hyperosmotic compared to beaker B.

(C) Beaker C is hypertonic and also hypo-osmotic compared to beaker A.

(D) Beaker A is hypotonic and hypo-osmotic compared to beaker B.

9. Which one of the following body fluid volumes can be measured directly?
   (A) Blood volume
   (B) Interstitial volume
   (C) Extracellular volume
   (D) Intracellular volume

ANSWERS AND EXPLANATIONS

1. **The answer is C.** A concentrated NaCl solution remains outside the cells because both Na^+ and Cl^- are excluded from the cells. Na^+ is removed from the cells by the Na^+–K^+-ATPase, and Cl^- equilibrates according to its electrochemical potential. This causes the osmotic movement of water from the cells into the extracellular spaces, and the intracellular volume decreases. Both the interstitial volume and the total extracellular volume increase. Because a solution has been infused, the total body water will increase. However, the distribution of the water between the compartments will change.

2. **The answer is A.** A 2 mmol/L solution will result in a 2 mmol/L concentration of Ca^{2+}. Because there are 2 mmol/L of Ca^{2+}, and the Ca^{2+} has two positive charges, there is a total of 4 mEq/L of Ca^{2+}. $CaCl_2$ breaks down into three particles when in solution. Therefore, there are three particles for each mmol. Because there are 2 mmol/L and three particles/mmol, there is a total of 6 mOsm/L. The mEq of Cl^- must be the same as the mEq of Ca^{2+}. The solution will yield 4 parts of Cl^-, each of which has one negative charge. Therefore, there are also 4 mEq/L of Cl^-.

3. **The answer is B.** A patient with severe renal failure will have an increased plasma creatinine concentration. The major route of elimination of creatinine from the body is through the kidneys. Loss of the ability to eliminate creatinine results in a continuous rise in plasma concentration. Loss of protein in the urine results in a decreased plasma protein concentration. It is the plasma protein concentration that determines the colloid osmotic pressure of the plasma and prevents the loss of plasma into the interstitium. Although a decreased plasma volume might, at first thought, lead to an increased RBC concentration, it is the kidney that is responsible for the release of erythropoietin and subsequent stimulation of RBC production by the bones. Loss of the ability to stimulate RBC production may even lead to a decrease in hematocrit. Similar to creatinine, the major route of K^+ elimination is by the kidneys. An inability to excrete K^+ in the urine leads to an increase in K^+ concentration, not a decrease.

4. **The answer is C.** An 80-kg individual would have a total body water of approximately 60% of his body weight, or 48 kg. Because 1 L of water weighs 1 kg, the total body water is 48 L. The plasma, the ECF, and the ICF must be in osmotic equilibrium. At the start of the baseball game there is a total of 14,400 mOsm (48 L × 300 mOsm/L). After losing 3 kg of water, there are 45 L of total body water. The new osmolarity is 14,400 mOsm/45 L, which equals 320 mOsm/L. The total body fluids will come to osmotic equilibrium at this value. If the loss were only from the extracellular volume (20% body weight), the osmolarity would be 369 mOsm/L (option A). If the loss were only from the intracellular volume (40% body weight), the osmolarity would be 331 mOsm/L (option B). If all the body were water (80 L), the answer would be 312 mOsm/L (option D). However, the body is not all water, and the total body water must come to osmotic equilibrium.

5. **The answer is B.** This is a two-part logic question. First, the volume of distribution must be determined, and then the appropriate compartment must be determined. Because 3 g of drug Z was injected, and 1 g was lost in the urine, there are 2 g of drug

Z left in the body. The final concentration in the plasma is 1 g/L (1 mg/mL = 1 g/L). Dividing the total amount left (2 g) by the final concentration (1 g/L) gives a volume of 2 L. What does this volume represent? In this 10-kg pediatric patient, 2 L is equivalent to 20% of body weight and is approximately equal to the extracellular volume.

6. **The answer is C.** Sweating results in a loss of hypo-osmotic fluid. The osmolarity of the fluid left in the body increases. Because the initial loss of water is from the extracellular volume, the osmolarity of the ECF tends to increase. However, before any appreciable increase occurs, water is removed from the intracellular compartment, and the intracellular volume also decreases. Ingestion of salt tablets increases the total osmolarity because of the addition of osmotic particles to the body. Because the Na^+ and Cl^- remain in the ECF, the increased osmolarity results in movement of water out of the intracellular space, and the volume of the intracellular space decreases until the osmolarity of both compartments is equal. Ingestion of excess water decreases the total body osmolarity by increasing the volume of both compartments. Most sports beverages have the same osmolarity as plasma and increase only the extracellular volume. Most of the osmotic particles are glucose, with a surprisingly small amount of electrolytes. In the absence of exercise, these drinks can be a significant source of excess calories. After the body metabolizes the glucose, what is left is essentially a very dilute fluid that increases the volume in both compartments and decreases total osmolarity.

7. **The answer is C.** An increase in the negative charge results in a greater attraction for the X^+ in compartment B. The X^+ molecules will move along the increased electrochemical gradient from compartment B to compartment A. Therefore, the concentration in compartment B will decrease, and the concentration in compartment A will increase. Obviously, the concentration difference between the two compartments will also increase. The movement of X^+ is due to the increased potential difference and·is not the cause of it.

8. **The answer is D.** Tonicity is referenced to the osmolarity of plasma, which is normally approximately 280 mOsm/L. A concentration less than plasma is hypotonic, whereas a concentration greater than plasma is hypertonic. Osmolarity is simply a comparison of the osmotic concentration between two solutions. Thus, beaker B has the same osmolarity as plasma and is isotonic. Because the osmolarity of beaker B is greater than beaker A, it is hyperosmotic compared to beaker A. Beaker C has a higher osmolarity than plasma and is therefore hypertonic. It is also hyperosmotic compared to both A and B. Beaker A has a lower osmolarity than plasma and is hypotonic. It is also hypo-osmotic to beaker B because the osmolarity is lower beaker than B.

9. **The answer is C.** Blood volume is a combination of both plasma volume and RBC volume. Interstitial volume must be calculated as the difference between plasma volume and extracellular volume, whereas intracellular volume is the difference between total body water and extracellular volume. Extracellular volume can be directly measured using radiolabeled Na^+.

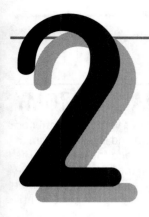

BASIC RENAL PROCESSES

CHAPTER OUTLINE

INTRODUCTION OF CLINICAL CASE

A healthy 25-year-old man presents to his physician for an evaluation prior to donating one kidney to his brother for transplantation. He then returns 1 month after removal of the kidney for a checkup. A comparison of major laboratory values before and 1 month after surgery is presented in Table 2-1.

◀ **TABLE 2-1**
Laboratory Values Before and 1 Month After Surgery

Value	Before Surgery	After Surgery	Normal
Serum			
Sodium	140 mEq/L	138 mEq/L	135–145 mEq/L
Potassium	4.0 mEq/L	4.2 mEq/L	3.8–5.1 mEq/L
Bicarbonate	24 mEq/L	24 mEq/L	23–29 mEq/L
Glucose	100 mg/dL	90 mg/dL	70–115 mg/dL
Creatinine	0.9 mg/dL	1.3 mg/dL	0.7–1.3 mg/dL
Urine			
Volume	1500 mL/24 hours	2000 mL/24 hours	Depends on intake
Sodium	100 mEq/L	80 mEq/L	Depends on intake
Potassium	70 mEq/L	55 mEq/L	Depends on intake
Bicarbonate	0 mEq/L	0 mEq/L	
Glucose	0 mg/dL	0 mg/dL	
Creatinine	100 mg/dL	75 mg/dL	Depends on muscle mass

BASIC RENAL ANATOMY

The renal mass can be divided into two primary regions; the cortex and medulla.

Fig. 2-1 provides an illustration of the major structures observed in a vertically sectioned human kidney, which typically measures less than 12 cm in length and less than 8 cm in width. The renal mass is divided into two major regions, the cortex and the medulla. The medulla can be further subdivided into an outer and inner zone. In the human kidney, the medulla is divided into multiple renal pyramids, each of which tapers to form a renal papilla. Notably, the number of papillae is species dependent, ranging from the multi-papillate human kidney to the unipapillate (single papilla) rat kidney. The inner core of the kidney is essentially a collecting chamber for urine (the pelvic space), which is created from an extension of the ureter. Each papilla projects into this pelvic space via the minor calices. The minor calices then converge into two or three chambers known as major calices. Finally, the major calices converge to form the pelvis, which represents the initial transition from the ureter as it enters the kidney via an indentation known as the hilus. The calices, renal pelvis, and ureters are surrounded by smooth muscle fibers, which force urine from the pelvis to the urinary bladder by peristaltic contractions.

FIGURE 2-1 ▶

Major Anatomic Structures Observed in a Vertically Sectioned Human Kidney.
Modified from Vander AJ: Renal Physiology, 4th ed., New York: McGraw-Hill, 1991, p. 7.

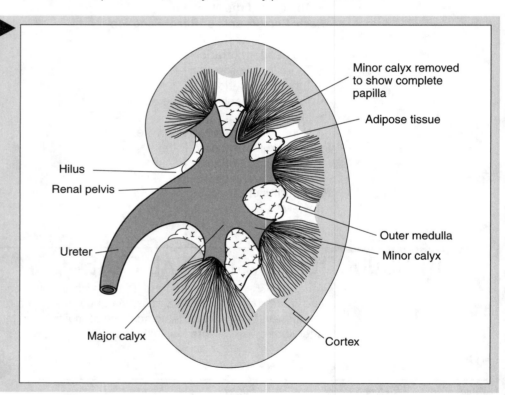

Minor calyx removed to show complete papilla

Adipose tissue

Hilus

Renal pelvis

Ureter

Outer medulla

Minor calyx

Major calyx

Cortex

Renal Vascular Arrangement

Unique vascular arrangement; afferent arteriole → glomerular capillaries → efferent arteriole → peritubular capillaries.

The renal artery also enters the renal mass via the hilum. As illustrated in Fig. 2-2, the renal artery then subdivides into a series of segmental (interlobar) arteries, each of which supplies a specific area of renal tissue. The interlobar arteries give rise to arcuate arteries from which a series of interlobular arteries ascend through the cortical mass toward the surface of the kidney. Multiple afferent arterioles branch off each interlobular artery, which themselves branch to form the glomerular capillaries. The glomerular capillaries reconverge to form efferent arterioles, which then branch once more to form an extensive peritubular capillary network. The vasa recta illustrated in Fig. 2-2 are specialized peritubular capillaries that arise exclusively from the efferent arterioles of so-called juxtamedullary nephrons (see below). Vasa recta exhibit a hairpin-loop configuration and provide the primary blood supply to the inner medulla. Although not shown on Fig. 2-2,

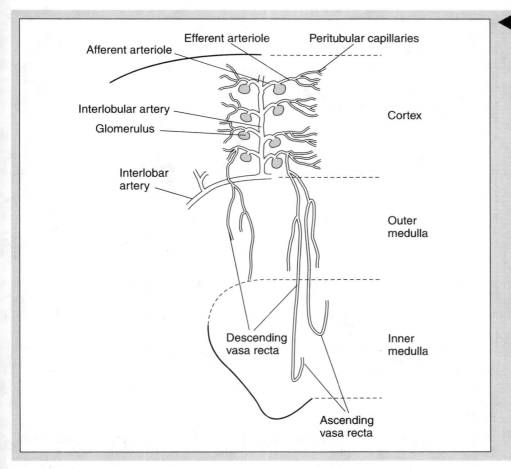

◀ **FIGURE 2-2**
Renal Vasculature. *For diagrammatic clarity, only the arterial side of this system is presented. The peritubular capillaries (including the vasa recta) ultimately reconverge to create a venous system that terminates in the renal vein. Modified from Koeppen BM, Stanton BA:* Renal Physiology, *St. Louis, MO: Mosby Yearbook, 1992, p. 58.*

the peritubular capillaries ultimately reconverge to create a renal venous system consisting sequentially of stellate → interlobular → arcuate → interlobar → renal veins.

An appreciation of this vascular arrangement provides a basis for understanding at least two important issues. First, there probably is considerably more available renal function than is actually required to maintain body fluid homeostasis. There are many instances of living family members donating kidneys for transplantation. These donors are able to survive perfectly normally with one kidney. In fact, people can survive with one kidney functioning at less than 100% capacity. Experimentally, this can be demonstrated simply by ligating selected interlobar arteries, which stops all blood flow, and thus all function, in a defined region of the kidney. Therefore, it is possible to assess the ability of an experimental subject to maintain fluid homeostasis after complete removal of one kidney and, for example, one-third nephrectomy of the remaining kidney.

A second important issue relates to the impact of this vascular arrangement on the blood pressure profile within the kidney. The kidney exhibits a very unique vascular sequence consisting of an afferent arteriole, glomerular capillary, and efferent arteriole. The afferent and efferent arterioles are, in fact, the two major sites of vascular resistance within the kidney. Their effects on the pressure profile of the renal vasculature are illustrated in Fig. 2-3. This unique pressure profile has major implications for at least two critical components of overall renal function. First, the process of glomerular filtration depends on the fact that, in contrast to other capillary beds, hydrostatic pressure along the length of the glomerular capillaries is high and remains relatively constant. Second, the extremely low residual hydrostatic pressure in the peritubular capillaries helps promote the process of tubular reabsorption, particularly along the proximal tubule.

Two kidneys provide a large degree of reserve functional capacity.

The afferent and efferent arterioles are the major sites of vascular resistance within the kidney.

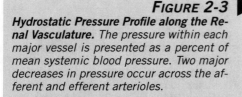

FIGURE 2-3

Hydrostatic Pressure Profile along the Renal Vasculature. *The pressure within each major vessel is presented as a percent of mean systemic blood pressure. Two major decreases in pressure occur across the afferent and efferent arterioles.*

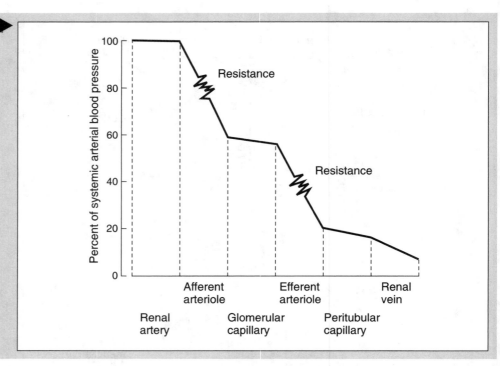

Anatomy of the Nephron

The functional unit of the kidney is the nephron. Human kidneys each contain approximately 1 million nephrons. Each nephron consists of two principal components, the glomerulus and the tubule. The glomerulus essentially consists of a bed of capillaries (the glomerular capillaries) contained within a terminal extension of the renal tubule known as Bowman's capsule. The renal tubule itself is a tube just one epithelial layer in thickness. The tubule can be subdivided into a series of functionally and morphologically distinct segments. The major subdivisions include the proximal tubule, the loop of Henle, the distal tubule, and the collecting tubule system (Fig. 2-4). Each of these major components, however, can be further subdivided, again based on both functional and morphologic criteria. For example, the proximal tubule traditionally has been subdivided into the proximal convoluted and proximal straight segment (the pars recta). More recently however, this nephron segment has been even further subdivided into so-called S_1 (early), S_2 (middle), and S_3 (late) components. The loop of Henle is comprised of a thin descending limb, a thin ascending limb (in a subset of nephrons; see below), and a thick ascending limb (in all nephrons). The thick ascending limb can be further subdivided into an outer medullary and a cortical segment. The distal tubule consists almost exclusively of a distal convoluted tubule but can also include a short connecting tubule that leads into the collecting tubule system. This final major component of the nephron is traditionally subdivided into a cortical, outer medullary, and inner medullary (or papillary) collecting tubule.

> *Each renal tubule is one epithelial cell layer thick.*

Although the above general description is representative of all nephrons, there are at least two anatomically and probably functionally distinct populations of nephrons within the kidney, based in part on the specific location of the glomerulus within the cortex (see Fig. 2-4). The glomeruli of superficial (or cortical) nephrons are typically located close to the surface of the kidney, whereas the glomeruli of juxtamedullary nephrons are located deeper in the cortex. Superficial nephrons have a loop of Henle, which typically descends no further than the junction between the inner and outer medulla; therefore, they often are referred to as "short-looped" nephrons. In contrast, the loop of Henle of juxtamedullary nephrons can descend well into the inner medulla. It is this subset of so-called "long-looped" nephrons that possesses a thin ascending limb of the loop of Henle. Juxtamedullary nephrons play a critical role in the process of urine concentration. The proportion of superficial to juxtamedullary nephrons is species dependent, with the human kidney typically consisting of 80% superficial nephrons.

> *Nephrons may be classified as superficial (cortical) or juxtamedullary.*

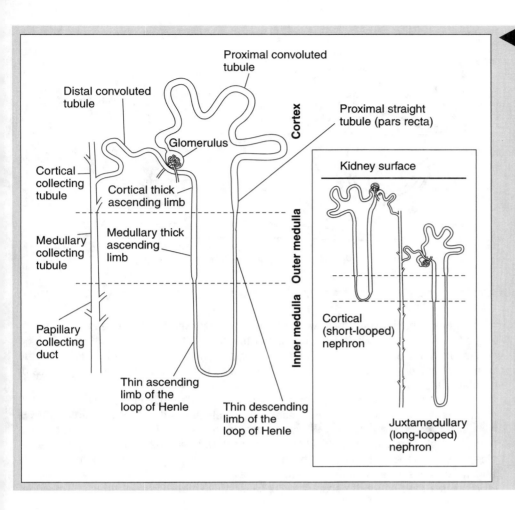

FIGURE 2-4
Functional Unit of the Kidney: The Nephron. Each nephron consists of two major components, the glomerulus and the tubule. The tubule can be subdivided into several functionally and, morphologically distinct segments. The small insert to the right emphasizes that at least two major subpopulations of nephrons exist, which are referred to as cortical ("short-looped") and juxtamedullary ("long-looped") nephrons.

BASIC COMPONENTS OF RENAL FUNCTION

As illustrated in Fig. 2-5, there are three primary components to renal function. The first is referred to as *glomerular filtration*, the process whereby an ultrafiltrate of plasma is transferred out of the circulatory system and into the renal tubule. The composition of this filtered fluid can then be modified by two fundamental processes. The first process, *tubular reabsorption*, is the process whereby water or solute is transported out of the tubular lumen and returned to the circulatory system, thereby preventing it from being excreted in the urine. The second process, *tubular secretion*, is the process whereby certain solutes can be transported into the tubular lumen from the peritubular capillaries, which are located downstream of the glomerulus. Tubular secretion therefore provides a mechanism for adding solutes to the tubular fluid, which is ultimately excreted as urine. It is the integrated effects of these three principal components of renal function—filtration, reabsorption, and secretion—that ultimately lead to the production and subsequent excretion of urine of precisely defined composition.

The three primary components of renal function: glomerular filtration, tubular reabsorption, and tubular secretion.

Magnitude of Renal Function

Typical values for overall renal function are quite remarkable. Although the two kidneys of an average person weigh only 300 g or so, they are perfused with approximately 1.5 L of blood per minute, which translates to approximately 25% of total cardiac output. On a per-gram basis, this means that the blood flow rate to the renal cortex is approximately 100 times higher than that of resting muscle. An appreciation of this very high blood flow rate also is important for explaining what at first glance may seem somewhat paradoxical. In contrast to other organs, the difference in oxygen content between the renal artery and

The kidneys receive approximately 25% of total cardiac output.

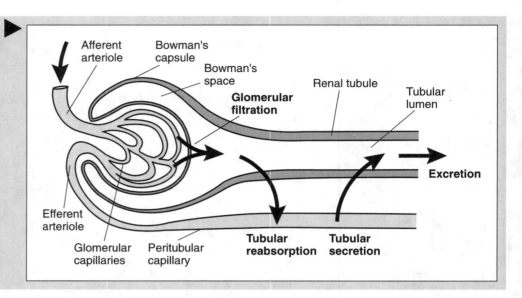

FIGURE 2-5

Major Components of Renal Function: Glomerular Filtration, Tubular Reabsorption, and Tubular Secretion.

Renal oxygen consumption is high and primarily required for tubular reabsorption.

Glomeruli filter approximately 180 L of fluid per day.

The actual amounts of water and solute excreted can be varied according to homeostatic demands.

The entire plasma volume is filtered and thus processed some 60 times each day, which helps prevent oscillations in body fluid volume and composition.

Fluid filtered by the glomerulus is essentially a protein-free ultrafiltrate of plasma.

The driving force for glomerular filtration is determined by the balance of Starling forces.

the renal vein is relatively small, which seemingly suggests that the oxygen requirement of the kidney is quite low. In fact, this is not the case. When the very high rate of blood flow is taken into account, oxygen *consumption* per unit time by the kidney is one of the highest of any organ. Much of this oxygen is absolutely required to fuel the process of tubular reabsorption.

Each day, the glomeruli filter approximately 180 L of fluid. Of that 180 L, only 1.5 L of fluid are typically excreted as urine each day, which means that 178.5 L (or 98% of the so-called "filtered load") are reabsorbed. Considering sodium ions (Na^+), it can be seen that although approximately 25,200 mEq are filtered each day (180 L/day filtered × plasma Na^+ concentration of 140 mEq/L), most of the Na^+ is reabsorbed because only 150 mEq or less are typically excreted in the urine. Glucose handling by the kidney represents a case of total reabsorption because this solute is freely filtered; yet under normal circumstances, no glucose appears in the urine.

Two important facts must be emphasized. First, the actual amounts of water and solute that are excreted are not fixed but rather can be varied according to homeostatic demands. As discussed in Chapter 1, input must be equal to output to maintain body fluid homeostasis. Therefore, 1.5 L of water are eliminated per day when there is a net intake of water to the body of 1.5 L/d. Similarly, if 150 mEq of Na^+ are consumed per day, then 150 mEq must be eliminated per day to maintain homeostasis. If intake changes, appropriate changes in excretion also occur. In most cases, this is achieved by altering the percentage of the filtered load that is reabsorbed. Second, maintenance of body fluid homeostasis depends on constant processing by the kidneys. The high rate of filtration ensures that this occurs. With a plasma volume of approximately 3 L, a glomerular filtration rate (GFR) of 180 L/day means that the entire plasma volume is filtered, and thus processed, 60 times each day. In contrast to the hemodialysis condition discussed in Chapter 1, frequent processing helps to prevent oscillations in body fluid volume and composition.

GLOMERULAR FILTRATION

Fluid filtered by the glomerulus is essentially a protein-free ultrafiltrate of plasma. As discussed in detail in Chapter 3, a combination of capillary endothelium, basement membrane, and tubular epithelium creates a permselective membrane, which impedes the filtration of larger, negatively charged solutes. Smaller substances (typically less than 5000 daltons) are freely filtered. Thus, the concentration of each of these solutes in the fluid in Bowman's space is essentially identical to that in plasma. Just as it is for the movement of fluid across extrarenal capillaries, the driving force for glomerular filtration is determined by the balance of Starling forces (Fig. 2-6). The situation in the glomerulus is slightly simplified, however. Because the glomerular capillary is essentially impermeable to protein, the colloid osmotic or oncotic pressure in Bowman's space can be considered to be zero. Therefore, net filtration pressure (NFP) is derived as follows:

$$NFP(mm\ Hg) = P_{GC} - P_{BS} - \pi_{GC}$$

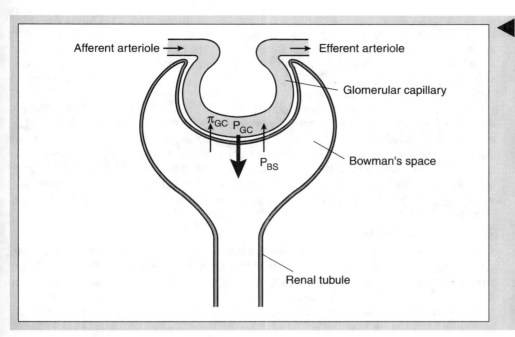

FIGURE 2-6
Impact of Starling Forces on Glomerular Filtration. The major driving force for filtration is the hydrostatic pressure within the glomerular capillaries (P_{GC}). Two forces oppose filtration, the hydrostatic pressure within Bowman's space (P_{BS}), and the colloid osmotic (oncotic) pressure within the glomerular capillaries (π_{GC}). Because plasma proteins are poorly filtered, the colloid osmotic pressure within Bowman's space is negligible. Modified from Vander AJ: Renal Physiology, 4th ed., New York: McGraw-Hill, 1991, p. 7.

where P_{GC} = hydrostatic pressure in the glomerular capillary, P_{BS} = hydrostatic pressure in Bowman's space, and π_{GC} = oncotic pressure in the glomerular capillary.

Under normal circumstances, the balance of these three forces generates a NFP of 10–15 mm Hg, a value that is comparable to the NFP at the arteriolar end of a systemic capillary. However, this NFP results in the movement of much more fluid across a glomerular capillary than across a systemic capillary. This is because an additional factor, the ultrafiltration coefficient (K_f) must be taken into consideration. The K_f is a function of both the water permeability of the capillary as well as the total surface area. Because the water permeability of glomerular capillaries is 100-fold higher than that of systemic capillaries, and capillary density is at least twofold higher, the K_f of glomerular capillaries is much greater than that of systemic capillaries.

One additional distinction should be made between glomerular and systemic capillaries. As presented in the *left panel* of Fig. 2-7, the balance of Starling forces favors net filtration across the first 50% of the systemic capillary because capillary hydrostatic pressure exceeds colloid osmotic pressure. The balance of Starling forces favors net reabsorption across the remaining 50% when colloid osmotic pressure exceeds capillary hydrostatic pressure. This dramatic shift occurs primarily as a result of the progressive drop in hydrostatic pressure along the length of the capillary. As can be seen in the *right panel* of Fig. 2-7, the

The K_f of glomerular capillaries is much greater than that of systemic capillaries.

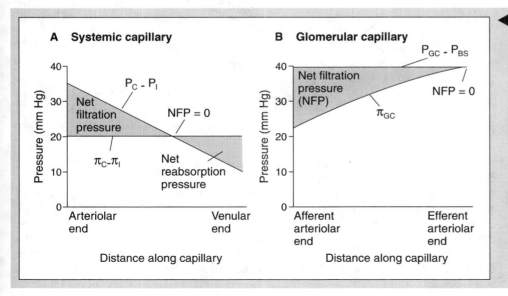

FIGURE 2-7
Comparison of the Impact of Starling Forces on Fluid Movement along the Length of Either (A) a Systemic Capillary or (B) a Glomerular Capillary. For the systemic capillary, symbols represent hydrostatic (P) and oncotic (π) pressures in the capillary (C) and interstitium (I) respectively. For the glomerular capillary, pressures in the glomerular capillary (GC) and Bowman's space (BS) are presented. Both net filtration and net reabsorption occur along systemic capillaries, primarily as a result of the progressive drop in capillary hydrostatic pressure that occurs along the length of the capillary. In contrast, hydrostatic pressure remains relatively constant along the length of the glomerular capillary, thereby helping to sustain a net pressure favoring filtration.

situation is very different in the glomerular capillary. Here, P_{GC} remains relatively constant along the entire length of the capillary. Consequently, the balance of Starling forces favors filtration until a point is reached where oncotic pressure within the glomerular capillary rises sufficiently such that $P_{BS} + \pi_{GC} = P_{GC}$. At this point, NFP is zero, and filtration ceases. In the example given, this point is achieved toward the end of the glomerular capillary. Beyond this point, no filtration (or reabsorption) occurs. Yet, how does P_{GC} remain relatively constant along the length of the glomerular capillary? The answer lies in the unique vascular arrangement surrounding the glomerular capillaries discussed earlier. Recall that there is a resistance vessel not only immediately upstream (the afferent arteriole) but also immediately downstream (the efferent arteriole) of the capillary bed. It is this downstream resistance point in particular that is critical to the maintenance of hydrostatic pressure within the glomerular capillaries. Using a garden hose analogy, recall how pressure within the hose increases upstream of an added resistance (e.g., a foot).

TUBULAR REABSORPTION

As described earlier, once fluid is filtered into the renal tubule, it must undergo selective processing to ultimately form urine. The process of tubular reabsorption affords an opportunity to remove water or solutes from this filtered fluid and return it to the circulation. As presented in Fig. 2-8, however, this seemingly simple process involves a series of coordinated steps. Recall that the renal tubule consists of a single layer of epithelial cells that are connected to each other by tight junctions. Most reabsorption

> P_{GC} remains relatively constant along the length of the glomerular capillary.

> Most reabsorption occurs transcellularly (through the cells), but some solutes can be reabsorbed paracellularly (between the cells).

FIGURE 2-8 ▶

A cross-section of a renal tubule illustrating the potential transcellular (through the cell) and paracellular (between the cells) routes of transepithelial transport of solutes and water from the tubular lumen into the peritubular capillary.

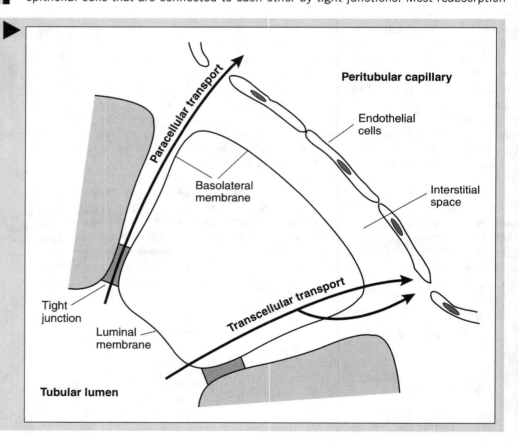

occurs through the cells (transcellularly) although, some solutes can be reabsorbed between the cells (paracellularly) via tight junctions (see Fig. 2-8). If the transcellular route is considered, reabsorption involves transport across two membranes—the luminal and basolateral membranes. The transport of most of the solutes across each membrane uses transport proteins, typically either a carrier protein or channel. Fig. 2-9 illustrates the transport systems involved in the reabsorption of Na$^+$ in the proximal tubule and the cortical collecting tubule. A critical element of this process common to both nephron segments is the presence of a Na$^+$–K$^+$-ATPase located exclusively on the basolateral membrane. This adenosine triphosphate (ATP)–driven pump extrudes Na^+ from the cell in exchange for potassium ions (K^+). The low intracellular Na^+ concentration in turn provides a favorable chemical gradient for Na^+ entry across the luminal membrane. However, the luminal transport process differs markedly in the two nephron segments. In the proximal tubule, Na^+ enters the cell via a Na^+–glucose cotransporter. In contrast, in the cortical collecting tubule, Na^+ enters the cell across the luminal membrane via an ion channel selective for Na^+. Therefore, the transport proteins do typically differ on the basolateral and luminal membranes, but these transporters work in concert to effect transcellular transport of solutes.

TUBULAR SECRETION

In essence, tubular secretion is the mirror image of reabsorption. The concerted action of transport proteins on the basolateral and luminal membranes enables selected solutes to be transported from the peritubular capillaries into the tubular lumen. Although reabsorption in one form or another occurs along the entire length of the nephron, tubular secretion is confined for the most part to the proximal tubule. Secretion of K^+ and hydrogen ions (H^+) are perhaps the two exceptions to this rule. What are these selected

Distinct basolateral and luminal membrane transporters work in concert to effect transcellular transport of solutes.

Tubular secretion is confined for the most part to the proximal tubule.

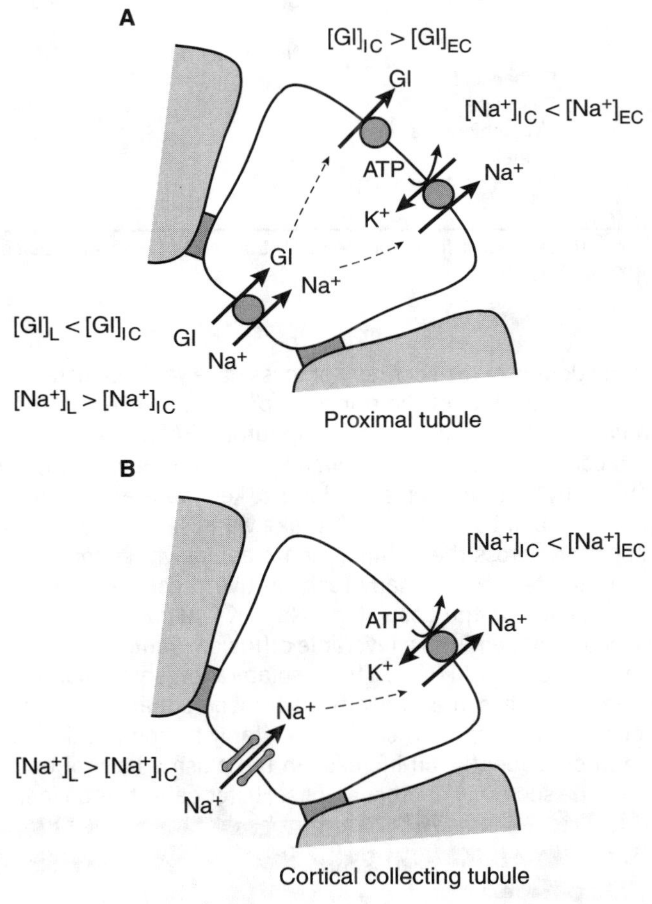

◀ **FIGURE 2-9**
Two examples of the mechanisms promoting transcellular reabsorption of Na^+. Note that in the proximal tubule, the movement of Na^+ across the luminal membrane occurs via a Na^+–glucose cotransporter (which is one example of a family of Na^+-coupled cotransporters), while in the cortical collecting tubule, Na^+ traverses the luminal membrane via a Na^+-selective ion channel. In both cells, the Na^+-K^+-ATPase is responsible both for the movement of Na^+ across the basolateral membrane, as well as for maintaining a favorable electrochemical gradient for luminal entry of Na^+. [] represents the concentration of either Na^+ or glucose (Gl) in the tubular lumen (L), intracellular fluid (IC) or extracellular fluid (EC).

solutes? Typically they are organic cations and anions (a partial listing of these solutes is given in Table 2-2). The critical importance of tubular secretion relates back to the permselectivity of the glomerulus (discussed above). Recall that both size and charge of a solute can markedly impede filtration. That being the case, how then can many large organic solutes be excreted? The answer is via secretion. In essence, secretion provides an opportunity to add a solute to the tubular fluid and, thus, allow the solute to be excreted. Interestingly, the efficacy of some clinically prescribed drugs depends on the secretory process. For example, the loop diuretic furosemide (Lasix) inhibits sodium chloride (NaCl) reabsorption in the thick ascending limb of the loop of Henle. Mechanistically, it directly inhibits the activity of a transport protein that is located exclusively on the luminal membrane of the cell. Consequently, it must be delivered to the loop of Henle via the tubular fluid. However, furosemide is not a readily filtered molecule, partly because it is bound to plasma proteins in the circulatory system. Consequently, the efficacy of furosemide depends on tubular secretion to deliver the drug to its site of action. This issue of protein binding can also affect the assessment of the renal handling of a number of substances. For example, the total plasma concentration of calcium (Ca^{2+}) is approximately 4 mEq/L. Consequently, one might anticipate a daily filtered load of Ca^{2+} of 720 mEq/d (180 L/d $\times$ 4 mEq/L). However, probably 50% of the total plasma Ca^{2+} is bound to plasma proteins and thus is unavailable for filtration. Consequently, a more likely filtered load is 360 mEq/d (180 L/d $\times$ 2 mEq/L) free Ca^{2+}.

TABLE 2-2 ▶

Examples of Substances Secreted by the Proximal Tubule

Endogenous Anions	Exogenous Anions	Endogenous Cations	Exogenous Cations
Cyclic adenosine monophosphate	Acetazolamide	Creatinine	Atropine
Bile salts	Chlorothiazide	Dopamine	Isoproterenol
Hippurates	Furosemide	Epinephrine	Cimetidine
Oxalate	Penicillin	Norepinephrine	Morphine
Prostaglandins	Probenecid		Quinine
Urate	Salicylate (aspirin)		Amiloride
	Hydrochlorothiazide		Procainamide
	Bumetanide		
	Para-aminohippuric acid		

Source: Reprinted with permission from Koeppen BM, Stanton BA: *Renal Physiology*, St. Louis, MO: Mosby Yearbook, 1992, p 58.

A number of the details of the secretory process have yet to be established; however, Fig. 2-10 provides a description of the transport proteins involved in the secretion of a typical organic anion, in this case para-aminohippurate (PAH). PAH is first taken up into the cell against its concentration gradient via a PAH-carboxylate antiporter. The di- and tri-carboxylates used by this antiporter include α-ketoglutate and glutarate, and are accumulated within the cell by basolateral uptake via a Na^+-carboxylate cotransporter. PAH is then transported across the luminal membrane down its concentration gradient via a PAH anion antiporter. As for many reabsorptive processes, secretion of organic anions ultimately depends on the basolateral Na^+–K^+-ATPase. In this case, the accumulation of carboxylates depends on a favorable diffusion gradient for Na^+, which in turn depends on the activity of this ATPase. The basolateral organic anion transporter has a low specificity; that is, it has the capacity to transport many different solutes. The functional impact of this fact is that there will inevitably be competition between solutes for the transporter. Consequently, an increase in the plasma level of one organic anion can adversely affect the secretion of other anions. Historically, this concept has been put to clinical use. Increased plasma PAH levels have been used to maintain more sustained plasma levels of penicillin by competing with this antibiotic for tubular secretory sites and, thus, retarding excretion.

TUBULAR TRANSPORT MAXIMUM

The renal tubule has a finite capacity to either reabsorb or secrete many solutes. The maximal transport capacity is referred to as the tubular transport maximum (T_m). The reason for this limitation is quite obvious because if transport depends on specific transport proteins, then once those transporters are fully occupied, no further increase in transport rate can occur. T_m values typically reflect the maximal transport capacity of both kidneys. This value in turn represents the sum of the transport capacities of all individual functional nephrons. It is worth noting that the T_m value of each nephron is probably not identical. Thus when the T_m of all individual nephrons has been exceeded, then the T_m of the kidneys is exceeded. The classic example to illustrate this concept is

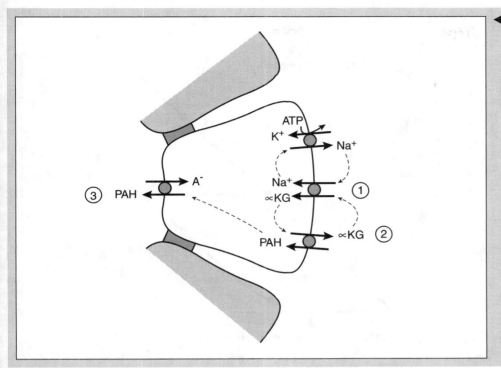

◀ **FIGURE 2-10**
Probable Mechanism Underlying the Secretion of Organic Anions (and Probably Cations) by the Proximal Tubule. In this model, para-aminohippurate (PAH) is the anion being transported. The process essentially consists of three sequential steps: 1. the transport of dicarboxylates such as α-ketoglutarate (α-KG) into the cell via a Na⁺-dependent cotransporter; 2. the transport of PAH into the cell via an α-KG-PAH antiporter; and 3. the transport of PAH into the lumen via a PAH-anion (A⁻) antiporter.

the renal handling of glucose, which is presented in Fig. 2-11. Under normal circumstances, no glucose is excreted in the urine, indicating that all filtered glucose must have been reabsorbed. With a normal plasma glucose concentration, therefore, the amount of glucose filtered is less than the T_m for glucose. Fig. 2-11 shows how glucose is handled as the filtered load is increased. To appreciate the T_m concept completely, three relatively simple calculations should be reviewed:

- Amount filtered (the filtered load): $GFR \times P_{Gl}$
- Amount excreted: $\dot{V} \times U_{Gl}$
- Amount reabsorbed: Amount filtered − amount excreted

where GFR = glomerular filtration rate, P_{Gl} = plasma glucose concentration, U_{Gl} = urine glucose concentration, and $\dot{V}$ = urine flow rate.

From the first formula, it can be appreciated that there are potentially two means of increasing the filtered load of glucose; either by progressive increases in the plasma concentration of glucose or by increasing GFR (or both). Experimentally, it is much easier to increase plasma glucose simply by infusion. Consequently, Fig. 2-11 illustrates the effects of increasing plasma glucose concentration on the amount filtered, the amount excreted, and, thus, the amount reabsorbed. As might be anticipated, a simple direct linear relationship exists between plasma glucose and the filtered load of glucose. Up to a certain filtered load, no glucose appears in the urine, indicating complete reabsorption. To this point, the lines representing amount filtered and amount reabsorbed are superimposeable. As we approach the T_m, glucose begins to appear in the urine, indicating that the reabsorptive capacity of some nephrons has been exceeded. With further increases in the filtered load, the T_m of progressively more nephrons is exceeded (the "splay"). Eventually, the T_m of all nephrons is exceeded, and at this point, reabsorptive capacity for glucose is maximal. Beyond this point, a direct linear relationship will therefore exist between the amount of glucose filtered and the amount excreted. The "threshold" value indicated on Fig. 2-11 represents the plasma glucose concentration at which glucose begins to appear in the urine (in other words, the concentration required to provide a filtered load of glucose that exceeds the T_m of at least some nephrons). It is important to understand that this is a derived and not a fixed number. For example, in Fig. 2-11, the threshold value is approximately 2 mg/mL. If the GFR were increased to 200 mL/min, a plasma glucose concentration of only 1 mg/mL would be required to achieve this same

The filtered load of a given solute can be altered by changes in the rate of glomerular filtration or the plasma concentration of the solute.

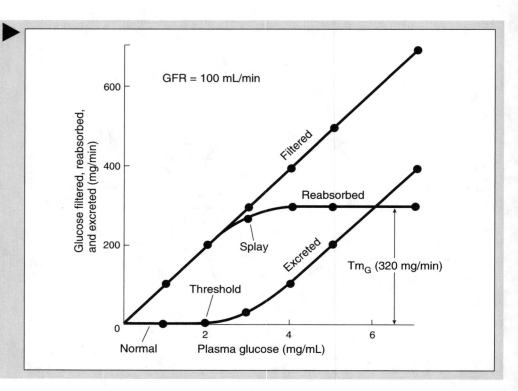

FIGURE 2-11

Tubular Transport Maximum for Glucose (Tm$_G$). *The amounts of glucose filtered, reabsorbed, and excreted (all expressed in mg/min) are plotted as a function of plasma glucose concentration (expressed in mg/mL). In this particular example, the glomerular filtration rate is held constant at 100 mL/min. The threshold value reflects the plasma glucose concentration at which glucose first appears in the urine.*

filtered load of 200 mg/min. Therefore, at that GFR, the plasma threshold would be 1 mg/mL. In the illustrated example, an even higher plasma glucose of approximately 3.2 mg/mL is required to present a filtered load of glucose that exceeds the T$_m$ for essentially all nephrons, which in this case is 320 mg/min.

In humans, the threshold value is much higher than normal plasma glucose concentrations. This implies that plasma glucose levels can rise considerably without the risk of losing this valuable fuel in the urine. A classic example of a situation when glucose does appear in the urine is diabetes mellitus. This is not a compensatory response but simply reflects the fact that the diabetes has caused the plasma glucose concentration to rise so high that the filtered load exceeds the T$_m$ for glucose.

Micturition

The urine that is formed by the renal tubules is ejected from the termini of the papillary collecting tubules directly into the renal pelvis. This urine passes down the ureters and is stored in the bladder prior to final elimination from the body. As described earlier, this movement of urine from the pelvis to the bladder is promoted by peristaltic contractions of the smooth muscle that surrounds the pelvis and the ureters. Parasympathetic innervation of these structures increases, and sympathetic innervation decreases this intrinsic contractility. The ureters also contain pressure receptors that are responsible for the sensation of intense pain that is associated with ureteral blockage caused by renal stones.

The bladder itself is composed of several layers of epithelial cells. It can be anatomically subdivided into the fundus, or body, and the neck, which connects the bladder to the urethra (Fig. 2-12). Most of the bladder is surrounded by a randomly distributed layer of smooth muscle fibers known as the detrusor muscle. At the bladder neck, however, a more orderly muscle fiber arrangement forms the so-called internal sphincter. The inherent tone in these fibers closes off the bladder neck during filling. The urethra is surrounded by a layer of skeletal muscle that is known as the external sphincter. Unlike the internal sphincter, the external sphincter is under voluntary control via the sympathetic pudendal nerve.

The average maximal capacity of the bladder is approximately 500 mL. As the bladder fills and nears capacity, internal pressure rises to the point where the so-called micturition reflex is activated. In this reflex, parasympathetic afferent nerves within the detrusor muscle layer detect the rise in pressure. This results in the activation of

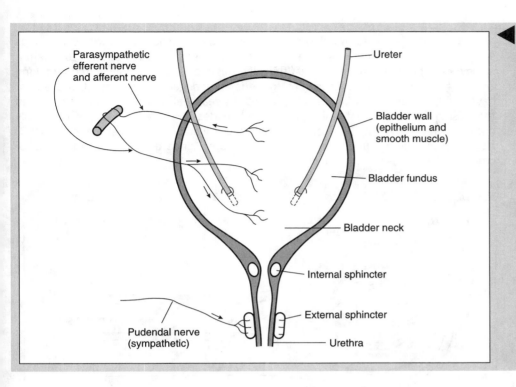

FIGURE 2-12
Basic Anatomy of the Urinary Bladder Including Parasympathetic and Sympathetic Innervation. *The area of the fundus at which the ureters enter the bladder is referred to as the trigone. Modified from Koeppen BM, Stanton BA:* Renal Physiology, *St. Louis, MO: Mosby Yearbook, 1992, p. 58.*

parasympathetic efferent nerve fibers that innervate the detrusor muscle and cause muscle contraction. The increased force of contraction eventually becomes strong enough to open the internal sphincter, which forces urine from the body of the bladder into the urethra. Voluntary relaxation of the external sphincter then permits final expulsion of the urine.

Noninvasive Assessment of Renal Function

GLOMERULAR FILTRATION RATE

The T_m concept discussed above has assumed that the GFR is known in this experimental subject. There are many disease processes that can adversely affect filtration (see Chapter 3); consequently, from a clinical perspective, it is important to be able to determine GFR. To determine GFR, a select group of substances that are handled by the kidney in a very specific fashion can be used. This group of substances includes inulin, sodium iothalamate, and creatinine. The essential characteristics of these compounds are:

The unique renal handling characteristics of substances such as inulin, sodium iothalamate and creatinine enable them to be used to estimate glomerular filtration rate.

• They are freely filterable
• They are not reabsorbed or secreted
• They are not produced or metabolized by the kidney
• They do not affect the GFR

Given these characteristics, it should be expected, based on a simple balance concept, that all of the inulin that is filtered per unit time (GFR $\times$ P_{IN}) will be equal to the amount excreted ($\dot{V} \times U_{IN}$) in the urine because this compound is neither reabsorbed or secreted (Fig. 2-13). Taking a little closer look at this formula:

$$GFR \times P_{IN} = \dot{V} \times U_{IN} \quad \text{and, rearranging,} \quad GFR = \frac{\dot{V} \times U_{IN}}{P_{IN}}$$

Then it becomes apparent that three easily attainable values can provide a reasonably accurate assessment of GFR. Urine flow rate can be determined by obtaining a timed urine collection, and inulin concentration in the voided urine and in a sample of plasma can be easily determined by colorimetric assay. The one disadvantage with compounds such as inulin or sodium iothalamate is that they must be infused initially to obtain a steady state plasma concentration. Clinically, this problem is circumvented by taking advantage of creatinine. Because creatinine is an endogenous compound, it does not have to be infused, and it is typically present at a reasonably constant concentration in the plasma. In reality, creatinine is, in fact, not an ideal GFR marker because it probably does undergo some tubular secretion that should lead to an overestimation of GFR. However, an inherent underestimation error in the standard analytical procedure for creatinine compensates for this overestimation.

FIGURE 2-13 ▶

Noninvasive Measurement of Glomerular Filtration Rate (GFR) using Inulin (IN). *Because inulin is neither reabsorbed nor secreted, the amount of inulin entering the nephrons (GFR × P_{IN}) should be equal to the amount leaving in the urine ($\dot{V} × U_{IN}$). P_{IN} = plasma concentration of inulin; U_{IN} = inulin concentration in urine; $\dot{V}$ = urine flow.*

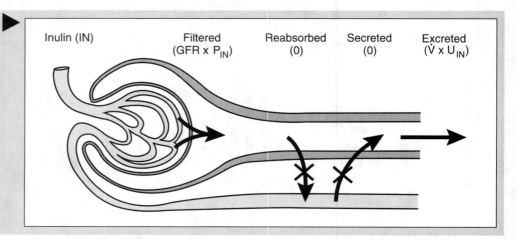

Inulin (IN)   Filtered ($GFR × P_{IN}$)   Reabsorbed (0)   Secreted (0)   Excreted ($\dot{V} × U_{IN}$)

RENAL PLASMA FLOW

Measurement of the clearance of PAH provides a non-invasive estimate of renal plasma flow.

This basic balance concept can be extended one step further to provide a method for the assessment of blood flow to the kidney. Obviously, the most direct way of doing this is to place a flow probe around the renal artery. However, in a clinical setting and in many experimental settings, this invasive procedure clearly is not practical. As above, the unique renal handling of selected compounds can be used to provide a measurement of renal plasma flow (RPF) noninvasively. The prototypic compound used in this analysis is PAH, which is an organic anion that is filtered to an extent but that is also secreted by the proximal tubule. Assuming that PAH is neither synthesized nor metabolized by the kidney, the balance concept predicts that all the PAH entering the kidney via the renal artery ($RPF_A × P_{PAH(A)}$) must be equal to the amount leaving the kidney in the renal vein ($RPF_V × P_{PAH(V)}$) and in the urine ($\dot{V} × U_{PAH}$). Again, looking a little more closely at this formula:

$$RPF_A × P_{PAH(A)} = (RPF_V × P_{PAH(V)}) + (\dot{V} × U_{PAH})$$

As stated previously, secreted substances are T_m limited just as reabsorbed substances are. Therefore, the reasonable assumption can be made that if the plasma concentration of PAH is kept below the level that would exceed the T_m, then all of the PAH that enters the kidney should be either filtered or secreted into the proximal tubule. On this basis, the concentration of PAH in the renal vein should be zero (Fig. 2-14). Consequently, the above formula becomes simplified to:

$$RPF_A × P_{PAH(A)} = \dot{V} × U_{PAH} \quad \text{and, rearranging,} \quad RPF_A = \frac{\dot{V} × U_{PAH}}{P_{PAH(A)}}$$

As in the case of measuring GFR, there is now a situation in which three easy measurements provide a reasonable estimate of RPF noninvasively. It should be emphasized that this provides only an estimate because PAH probably does not undergo complete removal from the plasma, consequently $P_{PAH(V)}$ is probably not zero. Therefore,

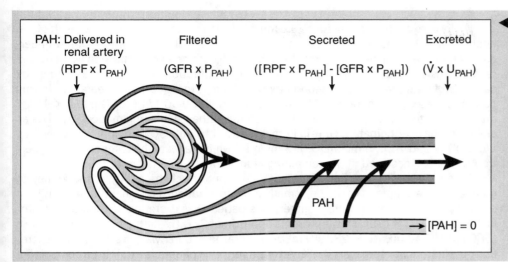

Noninvasive Measurement of Renal Plasma Flow (RPF) Using Para-Aminohippurate (PAH). *PAH is avidly secreted into the proximal tubule. Thus, if the plasma concentration of PAH is maintained below its transport maximum, the amount of PAH exiting the kidney via the renal vein should be zero. Under these conditions, then, all PAH entering the kidney in the renal artery ($RPF \times P_{PAH}$) should be equal to the amount leaving in the urine ($\dot{V} \times U_{PAH}$).*

this procedure more appropriately provides a measure of so-called effective renal plasma flow (ERPF). This value then can be taken one step further to provide an estimate of effective renal blood flow by taking into consideration the hematocrit (Hct), that is:

$$RBF = RPF / (1 - Hct)$$

CLEARANCE CONCEPT

The common features of the formula used to calculate GFR as well as RPF are used in the clearance formula, which provides a somewhat conceptual view of renal function expressed in units of volume and time. It was established above in the GFR calculation that all of the inulin contained within the volume of plasma that was filtered will be excreted in the urine. Almost all of the fluid, however, will be reabsorbed, thereby creating a "virtual volume" of plasma that is free of inulin. In other words, the volume of plasma that is equal to GFR has been "cleared" of inulin. Using the same reasoning, all of the PAH contained within the plasma that enters the kidney per unit time is also excreted in the urine. In this case, then, a volume of plasma equivalent to RPF is "cleared" of PAH. In summary, the "clearance" of, for example, inulin (C_{IN}) or creatinine (C_{CR}) is synonymous with GFR, whereas the "clearance" of PAH (C_{PAH}) is synonymous with RPF.

The clearance concept can be taken one step further to obtain some idea of how a particular substance (substance S) is handled by the renal tubules. Experimentally, if the clearance of inulin and the clearance of substance S are measured simultaneously, then the following conclusions can be drawn from the ratio of C_{IN}/C_S:

- If $C_{IN}/C_S > 1$, then net reabsorption of S must have occurred; in essence, reabsorbed S decreases the "virtual volume" of plasma cleared of S by filtration.
- If $C_{IN}/C_S < 1$, then net secretion of S must have occurred; in essence, further removal of S from the plasma by secretion increases the apparent size of this "virtual volume" of plasma.

RESOLUTION OF CLINICAL CASE

The first two chapters have emphasized the critical role the kidneys play in maintaining body fluid homeostasis. Consequently, it is reasonable to anticipate that removal of one kidney could have a major impact on the ability of an individual to maintain this homeostasis. As illustrated by the laboratory values, however, this is not the case. With the possible exception of plasma creatinine, both serum and urinary values are still well within their respective normal ranges after the nephrectomy, reinforcing the concept that people do possess considerable renal functional reserve capacity.

A closer examination illustrates a number of changes that occurred as a result of the nephrectomy. Perhaps the most pronounced change is that the remaining kidney undergoes compensatory hypertrophy, resulting in overall enlargement of the kidney, increased renal perfusion, and increased GFR. The change in filtration rate can be determined by calculating total pre- and postnephrectomy GFR from the creatinine clearance. In this particular case, prenephrectomy GFR is approximately 166 L/d (1500 mL/d × 1 mg/mL/0.009 mg/mL). At 1 month postnephrectomy, rather than being reduced by 50% as one might have anticipated, GFR is in fact reduced by only 30% to approximately 115 L/d (2000 mL/d × 0.75 mg/mL/0.013 mg/mL), which reflects the compensatory hypertrophy that has occurred in the remaining kidney over this period of time.

This reduced level of filtration clearly does not affect the ability of the kidney to maintain, for example, a normal plasma Na^+ concentration. The renal tubular handling of Na^+ changes however. Before surgery this patient was excreting 150 mEq/d of Na^+ (1.5 L/d × 100 mEq/L). This represents approximately 0.6% of the filtered load of Na^+ (166 L/d × 140 mEq/L = 23,240 mEq/d). Phrased another way, the "fractional excretion" of Na^+ prior to surgery is 0.6%. After surgery, this patient is excreting a comparable amount of Na^+ (160 mEq/d). However, the filtered load of Na^+ is considerably lower due to the reduced GFR and slightly lower serum Na^+ concentration (115 L/d × 138 mEq/L = 15,870 mEq/d). Thus, the fractional excretion of Na^+ has almost doubled to 1% after surgery (160/15,870 × 100%). In other words, the absolute renal tubular reabsorption of Na^+ has been reduced to compensate for the reduced filtered load.

With regard to the T_m concept, it should be apparent that the T_m for glucose is reduced after nephrectomy because the total number of nephrons, and thus total reabsorptive capacity, is reduced. However, glucose still does not appear in the urine because the filtered load of glucose is also much reduced and remains below the new T_m. Additionally, the plasma threshold value is not different after nephrectomy because both the T_m and filtered load, which determine the threshold value, have changed.

Finally, as was mentioned earlier, the plasma concentration of creatinine has increased as a result of the nephrectomy. For a substance such as creatinine, a steady-state plasma level is achieved when the rate of excretion is equal to the rate of production. In this case, it is known from the presented laboratory values that prior to the nephrectomy the rate of creatinine production was 1500 mg/d (the reported rate of excretion). Because creatinine is neither reabsorbed nor secreted, the filtered load of creatinine also must be 1500 mg/d. After the nephrectomy, the ability to excrete creatinine is impaired because GFR is reduced. Consequently, plasma creatinine concentration must increase, and it continues to do so until the filtered load once again reaches 1500 mg/d. In this case, at a GFR of 115 L/d, this occurs when plasma creatinine rises to 1.3 mg/dL.

REVIEW QUESTIONS

Directions: For each of the following questions, choose the **one best** answer.

1. Which one of the following statements is correct?
    - **(A)** The kidneys receive approximately 5% of cardiac output.
    - **(B)** Renal oxygen consumption must be low because the renal arteriovenous oxygen difference is small.
    - **(C)** Renal blood flow is equally distributed to the cortex and medulla.
    - **(D)** The kidney contains two types of capillary beds.

2. An individual has a T_m for glucose of 400 mg/min and an inulin clearance of 100 mL/min. What is the approximate plasma threshold for glucose in this individual?

    (A) 0.04 mg/mL

    (B) 0.4 mg/mL

    (C) 4 mg/mL

    (D) 40 mg/mL

3. Which one of the following substances has the lowest clearance in the human kidney?

    (A) Creatinine

    (B) Glucose

    (C) Potassium ion

    (D) Chloride ion

    (E) Para-aminohippuric acid (PAH)

4. Which one of the following statements is correct?

    (A) A steady-state plasma concentration of inulin is required to obtain an accurate estimate of glomerular filtration rate (GFR).

    (B) The absence of plasma substance X in the urine can only be because of the fact that it is not filtered.

    (C) Assuming that substance X is freely filterable, if $C_X < C_{IN}$, then X must be exclusively reabsorbed.

    (D) The fractional excretion of substance X should decrease if the reabsorption of X is decreased.

5. Which one of the following groups includes the proper items required to calculate renal plasma flow (RPF) rate at the beginning of the efferent arteriole?

    (A) Urine flow rate, urine para-aminohippuric acid (PAH), plasma PAH, urine inulin and plasma inulin concentrations

    (B) Urine flow rate, urine concentration of glucose, plasma concentration of glucose

    (C) Urine flow rate, urine concentration of glucose, plasma concentration of glucose

    (D) Urine flow rate, total osmolar clearance

6. Tubular secretion of organic anions is best described by which one of the following statements?

    (A) It occurs almost exclusively in the proximal tubule.

    (B) It is essential for excretion because organic anions cannot be filtered.

    (C) It is not a T_m-limited process.

    (D) It requires an ATP-dependent pump located on the luminal membrane.

ANSWERS AND EXPLANATIONS

1. **The answer is D.** The kidney contains glomerular capillaries that are enclosed within Bowman's capsules as well as peritubular capillaries that surround the renal tubules. The kidneys receive approximately 25% of the cardiac output, which translates to 1.5 L of blood per minute. It is true that the renal arteriovenous oxygen concentration difference is relatively small. However, renal blood flow is very high. Therefore, although oxygen extraction per unit volume of blood is low, the total amount extracted and subsequently consumed per unit of time is high. This oxygen is essential for maintaining the transport function of the kidney, and in particular for sustaining Na^+-K^+-ATPase activity. The renal cortex actually receives almost 90% of the blood delivered to the kidney.

2. **The answer is C.** By definition, the plasma glucose threshold is the plasma concentration at which glucose first appears in the urine. To excrete glucose, the filtered load must exceed the tubular transport maximum. In this individual, the T_m for glucose is 400 mg/min. Because the filtered load is calculated from $GFR \times P_{GL}$, and GFR (inulin clearance) is 100 mL/min, a plasma glucose concentration (P_{GL}) of 4 mg/mL is required to generate a filtered load of 400 mg/min. Recall that the stated T_m is actually an average value for all nephrons in the kidney. Because some nephrons will have a T_m that is lower than 400 mg/min, a filtered load of glucose that is equal to the average T_m will exceed the T_m of this subpopulation of nephrons, and thus will lead to glucose appearing in the urine.

3. **The answer is B.** Under normal circumstances, the clearance of glucose is actually zero. Because all of the filtered glucose is typically reabsorbed (and thus returned to the extracellular fluid compartment), the volume of plasma from which glucose is completely cleared per unit time is zero. At the other extreme, the highest possible clearance value is reflected in the clearance of PAH (option E). PAH is filtered and avidly secreted; as long as the T_m is not exceeded, the volume of plasma from which PAH is completely cleared per unit time is equivalent to the renal plasma flow. The clearances of creatinine, K^+, and Cl^- fall between these two extremes.

4. **The answer is A.** The clearance formula for calculating GFR assumes that the plasma concentration of the marker remains relatively constant during the period of urine collection. For an exogenous compound such as inulin, this is accomplished by maintaining a constant infusion of inulin throughout the experiment. If substance X does not appear in the urine, there are three possibilities: it is not filtered, it is not secreted, or, as is the case for glucose, all that is filtered is completely reabsorbed. It is true that reabsorption must have occurred for the clearance of substance X to be less than the clearance of inulin. However, it cannot be determined from this ratio that X has been *exclusively* reabsorbed by the renal tubule. The clearance of K^+ is typically less than that of inulin, yet K^+ is both reabsorbed and secreted by the tubule. In other words, this ratio provides an estimate of the overall handling of a given substance by the kidney. Therefore, under the conditions in option C, it can be said that *net* reabsorption of X has occurred, but not that X has been *exclusively* reabsorbed. The fractional excretion of X is the amount excreted divided by the amount filtered. If the reabsorption of X is selectively decreased, then the amount excreted must increase, and thus the fractional excretion will increase.

5. **The answer is A.** Because the efferent arteriole is downstream of the glomerular capillaries, plasma flow at this point must be equivalent to the volume entering the kidney in the renal artery (i.e., RPF rate) minus the volume of plasma that is filtered by the glomeruli (i.e., GFR). The options provided enable one to arrive at the same answer with a more extensive set of calculations. In this case, a combination of urine flow rate, urine para-aminohippuric acid (PAH) concentration, and plasma PAH concentration may be used to calculate effective RPF, and a combination of urine flow rate, urine inulin concentration, and plasma inulin concentration can be used to calculate GFR using standard clearance formulae.

6. **The answer is A.** Tubular secretion occurs almost exclusively in the proximal tubule only when referring to organic anions and cations. For example, both K^+ and H^+ are secreted by nephron segments other than the proximal tubule. Many organic anions, such as para-aminohippuric acid (PAH) are partially filterable. The reabsorption of many substances is T_m limited. This maximum reabsorptive capacity is fundamentally due to the fact that there is a finite number of transport proteins per cell to facilitate this reabsorptive process. Thus, when all transporters are fully saturated, the rate of reabsorption is maximal. Exactly the same principal applies to the process of secretion, which also depends on the presence of transport proteins in both the basolateral as well as the luminal membrane. Therefore, the secretion of organic anions is indeed a T_m-limited process. It is correct that the process of secretion does require the Na^+–K^+-ATPase. However, as is the case for all renal tubular cells, this pump is located exclusively on the *basolateral* membrane.

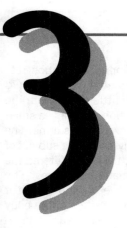

REGULATION OF GLOMERULAR FILTRATION RATE

CHAPTER OUTLINE

INTRODUCTION OF CLINICAL CASE

Mr. Smith, an 80-kg man with a history of hyperlipidemia, had been taking furosemide (a loop diuretic) for hypertension. He complained of headaches and generally did not feel well. His blood pressure was 150 mm Hg systolic and 105 mm Hg diastolic. A plasma sample was collected, and the following values were obtained: sodium (Na^+), 145 mEq/L (normal); potassium (K^+), 4.5 mEq/L (normal); creatinine, 1.5 mg/dL (slightly elevated); bicarbonate (HCO_3^-), 20.4 mEq/L (normal); and angiotensin II, 15 ng/mL/hr (high).

Mr. Smith was subsequently given an angiotensin-converting enzyme (ACE) inhibitor twice daily to inhibit the conversion of angiotensin I to angiotensin II. He returned 1 month later and felt worse than ever with lethargy and some edema. His sitting blood pressure was normal (115 mm Hg systolic and 75 mm Hg diastolic). A plasma sample was taken again with the following results: Na^+, 133 mEq/L (low); K^+, 6.0 mEq/L (high); creatinine, 6.5 mg/dL (high); HCO_3^-, 15.5 mEq/L (low); and angiotensin II, 0.5 ng/mL/hr (low).

MAGNITUDE OF GLOMERULAR FILTRATION

In a healthy individual, approximately 20%–25% of the resting cardiac output flows through the kidneys (see Chap. 2). In the "normal" 70-kg person, this represents a rate in excess of 1.2 L/min. Of this 1.2 L of blood, approximately 10% is filtered as protein-free plasma across the glomerular capillaries. Thus, the normal glomerular filtration rate (GFR) of approximately 120 mL/min or 180 L/d represents a substantial volume of fluid and electrolytes potentially lost from the circulation. In fact, very little is lost from the body. Most of the fluid and electrolytes are returned to the circulation, and only a small portion of the filtered fluid (typically 1.5 L/d) and electrolytes are excreted as urine. The control systems that regulate tubular transport of fluid and electrolytes are the subject of much of the remainder of this book. If the kidneys filter 180 L/d, they have filtered the entire volume of plasma in the cardiovascular system approximately 60 times. The functional significance of filtering and processing this large volume of fluid is that it provides a mechanism for precisely controlling the volume and composition of the body fluids. For example, despite large daily variations in Na+ intake, the plasma Na+ concentration typically varies less than 1% on a day-to-day basis as a result of this continuous processing of the filtered plasma. Although individuals may vary, the plasma Na+ concentration in any individual varies very little. At the other extreme, recall from Chap. 1 what happens when the daily function of the kidney must be replaced intermittently by artificial means (e.g., dialysis). Life is sustained, but there are large changes in body fluid volumes and composition between treatments.

> *The kidney filters the plasma volume approximately 60 times every day.*

> *The kidney maintains precise control over the body fluid volume and composition by processing and returning most of the filtered plasma to the body.*

THE GLOMERULUS

The glomerulus is technically the beginning of each individual nephron in the kidney. It consists of a set of glomerular capillaries contained within Bowman's capsule at the beginning of the proximal tubule. Blood flows into the glomerular capillaries through the afferent arteriole and exits the capillaries through the efferent arteriole. These arterioles are the major resistance vessels in the kidney and form what is known as a series circulation. The glomerulus is the site in the kidney where the plasma is filtered before it is processed by the tubules. The loss of the ability to filter plasma is the cause of diminished renal function in most patients with renal disease. It is necessary to have an understanding of the pressures in the glomerular capillary, the influence of the resistance vessels, and the nature of the impediments to filtration before discussing the factors which regulate GFR.

Glomerular Capillary Dynamics

It should be appreciated from Chap. 2 that the formation of glomerular filtrate is the result of physical forces that act at the glomerular capillaries. This relationship can be expressed for the glomerular capillary exactly the same way it is expressed for any capillary system:

Filtered fluid = permeability x area x [(capillary hydrostatic pressure - tissue

hydrostatic pressure) - (capillary oncotic pressure - tissue oncotic pressure)]

In the glomerular capillary, this can be expressed mathematically as:

$$GFR = K_f[(P_{GC} - P_{BS}) - (\pi_{GC} - \pi_{BS})]$$

where K_f = ultrafiltration coefficient (permeability × surface area of glomerular capillary); P_{GC} = hydrostatic pressure in glomerular capillary; P_{BS} = hydrostatic pressure in Bowman's space; π_{GC} = colloid osmotic pressure in glomerular capillary; and π_{BS} = colloid osmotic pressure in Bowman's space. Because virtually no protein crosses the glomerular capillary, π_{BS} is essentially 0.

The results of changes in physical pressures are fairly straightforward, and all pressures affect GFR. However, the glomerular capillary hydrostatic pressure (P_{GC}) is the one that can be physiologically controlled by the renal arterioles and therefore impacts GFR to the greatest extent. As an example, afferent arteriolar constriction upstream from the glomerular capillary would lead to a decrease in the glomerular capillary pressure and a decreased filtration of fluid from the capillary. GFR would thus decrease. Pathologic conditions also can lead to changes in pressures across the glomerular capillary. A kidney

> *GFR is determined by the pressures across the glomerular capillaries.*

stone or tubular obstruction that leads to increased pressure in Bowman's space (P_{BS}) would impede the filtration of fluid from the capillary and decrease GFR. Conversely, liver disease could result in decreased plasma protein concentration that would decrease capillary colloid osmotic pressure (π_{GC}) and be expected to result in an increased filtration rate. Lastly, an increase in the ultrafiltration coefficient (K_f) might be expected to increase filtration rate.

Series Arteriolar Resistance

The glomerular capillaries are located between two resistance arterioles—the afferent arteriole and the efferent arteriole. Increased resistance in either arteriole would decrease renal blood flow (RBF) because the arterioles are in series. However, a selective increase in resistance in either arteriole would have divergent effects on GFR. For instance, as stated earlier an increase in resistance at the afferent arteriole decreases blood flow and decreases glomerular capillary pressure by preventing blood flow into the glomerular capillary. Because glomerular capillary pressure is a major determinant of the filtration rate, GFR is decreased. Similar to the afferent arteriole, an increase in efferent arteriole resistance also decreases blood flow. However, by decreasing flow out of the glomerular capillary, the glomerular capillary pressure increases. Despite the decreased blood flow, GFR tends to increase. A useful analogy to illustrate this relationship is shown in Fig. 3-1. Imagine a flexible rubber tube with saltwater flowing through it. At two points on the tube are resistors, which represent the afferent and the efferent arterioles. Between the two resistors is a segment of tube with a hole representing the glomerular capillary from which fluid is pushed. Flow out of the tube is analogous to RBF (see Fig. 3-1A). Constriction of the afferent resistor (see Fig. 3-1B) decreases the outflow from the tube; it also decreases pressure downstream (P_{GC}) so that less fluid is forced out of the hole. Conversely, constriction of the efferent resistor (see Fig. 3-1C) also decreases the outflow from the tube. However, this also increases pressure upstream (P_{GC}), which forces more fluid out of the hole. Thus, from this analogy it can be seen that changes in afferent resistance have directionally similar effects on GFR and RBF, whereas changes in efferent resistance have directionally opposite effects on GFR and RBF. It should also be appreciated from the analogy that the composition of fluid pushed out of the hole is the same as the salty fluid flowing through the tube. Changes in the volume of fluid pushed out of the hole result in changes in both the volume of water and the amount of solute that are expelled from the tube.

Changes in afferent resistance change GFR and RBF in the same direction. Changes in efferent resistance have divergent effects on GFR and RBF.

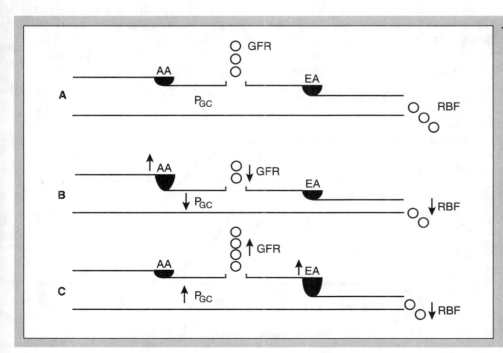

◀ **FIGURE 3-1**
Schematic Relationships among Afferent Arteriole (AA), Glomerular Filtration Rate (GFR), Efferent Arteriole (EA), Pressure in Glomerular Capillaries (P_{GC}), and Renal Blood Flow (RBF). (A) Normal conditions. (B) Increased resistance at AA decreases downstream pressure, GFR, and RBF. (C) Increased resistance at EA increases upstream pressure and GFR but decreases RBF.

Glomerular Capillary Permselectivity

Fluid is filtered at the glomerulus through a complex structure that consists of a capillary endothelial layer, a glomerular basement membrane, and an epithelial podocyte layer (Fig. 3-2). It is this complex structure that represents the barrier to fluid filtration by the glomerular capillaries. There are several differences between the glomerular capillary complex and systemic capillaries. First, despite the complexity of the glomerular capillaries, the permeability to water and electrolytes is much greater in the glomerular capillaries than in the systemic capillaries. Second, the glomerular capillary is only freely permeable to molecules with a molecular weight less than 5000 daltons. Finally, the glomerular capillary complex has a net negative charge.

FIGURE 3-2 ▶

Schematic Representation of the Glomerular Capillary Complex Illustrating the Capillary Endothelium, the Basement Membrane, and the Epithelial Podocytes. The foot processes represent points of attachment of the podocytes to the basement membrane.

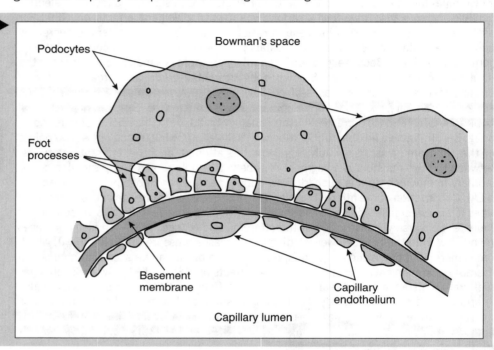

As pointed out above, the colloid osmotic pressure in Bowman's space is essentially 0 because almost no protein is filtered across the glomerular capillary. It is the negative charge on the glomerular capillary complex that is responsible for the inability of large, negatively charged protein molecules to cross the glomerular capillaries. They are repelled by the negative charge on the glomerular capillary complex. Fig. 3-3 shows the effect

The glomerular capillary complex has a net negative charge, which prevents the filtration of large negatively charged molecules such as albumin.

FIGURE 3-3 ▶

Effect of Size and Charge on the Molecular Permeability of the Glomerular Capillary. Very large negative molecules are less permeable than uncharged molecules. Na^+ = sodium; Cl^- = chloride; Suc = sucrose; UPP = uncharged polypeptide; PPP^+ = positively charged polypeptide; NPP^- = negatively charged polypeptide; In = inulin; Myo^- = myoglobin; Hb^- = hemoglobin; Alb^- = albumin.

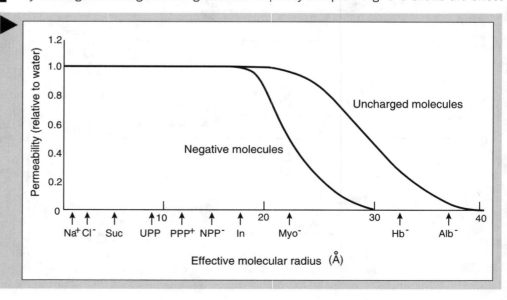

of molecular size and charge on the permeability of molecules relative to the permeability of water in the glomerular capillary. As can be seen, there is no effect of charge on the permeability of small molecules. However, in the case of large molecules, the permeability of negatively charged molecules is less than the permeability of similarly sized, uncharged molecules. Thus, the capillary displays *permselectivity* because the permeability of large charged molecules is based on size as well as charge.

Although there is relatively little protein filtered by the kidney under normal conditions, the patient with chronic renal failure presented in Chap. 1 had a low plasma albumin concentration, edema, and a large protein excretion in the urine. A very common clinical finding in advanced renal disease is a marked decrease in GFR concomitant with the loss of large amounts of albumin in the urine. Glomerular damage is the cause of both observations. Loss of the number of functioning glomeruli leads to decreased GFR, whereas loss of integrity of the remaining glomeruli leads to loss of the negative charge. The negatively charged albumin then behaves as an uncharged molecule, and the permeability to albumin increases, which leads to increased filtration of albumin. Thus, albumin appears in the urine. The loss of albumin leads to decreased systemic plasma colloid osmotic pressure and loss of fluid from the plasma volume into the interstitial space. Loss of fluid from the cardiovascular volume is the reason for the edema. The presence of low plasma protein caused by the abnormal loss of protein in the urine has been termed *nephrotic syndrome*.

The loss of negative charge on the glomerulus allows the filtration of negatively charged albumin molecules.

It should be appreciated that only a small increase in permeability to albumin is required to result in rather large increases in filtered albumin. In a healthy individual, the GFR is approximately 180 L/d, and the albumin concentration is approximately 45 g/L. If albumin were only 0.5% as permeable as water, it would take only 1 day to filter and excrete more than 40 g of albumin, which is almost equivalent to the amount of albumin in 1 L of plasma. Because the renal tubules have a very limited capacity to reabsorb filtered protein, it is easy to see how a large quantity of the filtered protein would be excreted in the urine. The liver may try to manufacture protein to compensate, but it has difficulty keeping up with the continuous loss.

INTRINSIC REGULATION OF GLOMERULAR FILTRATION RATE

In healthy individuals GFR normally changes very little. However, there are many everyday conditions that could potentially alter GFR. For instance, going from a supine to an upright position can increase blood pressure at the level of the kidneys. Similarly, the stress of an examination can increase blood pressure. Both situations tend to increase glomerular capillary pressure and increase GFR. It is easy to see that in the absence of a change in transport, an increase of only 10% in the GFR could cause an additional 18 L/d of plasma to be filtered and result in an inappropriate loss of fluid in the urine. Similarly, a decrease of 10% could result in the absence of urine output. How then does the kidney adjust for circumstances that could inappropriately change GFR? In fact, the kidney has the intrinsic ability to maintain a constant GFR under a variety of conditions. This ability to automatically regulate GFR at a constant value has been termed *renal autoregulation*.

*The kidney has the intrinsic ability to prevent spontaneous changes in GFR. This ability has been termed **renal autoregulation**.*

It has been found in the isolated, pump-perfused kidney that there are intrinsic renal mechanisms for maintaining GFR constant over a wide range of blood pressures. Fig. 3-4 shows the typical relationship between GFR as a function of renal artery perfusion pressure. When blood pressure increases above approximately 70 mm Hg, GFR remains reasonably constant. It can also be seen that when perfusion falls below about 70 mm Hg, GFR changes directly with changes in perfusion pressure. The pressure below which the kidney can no longer autoregulate GFR has been termed the *threshold* for *autoregula-*

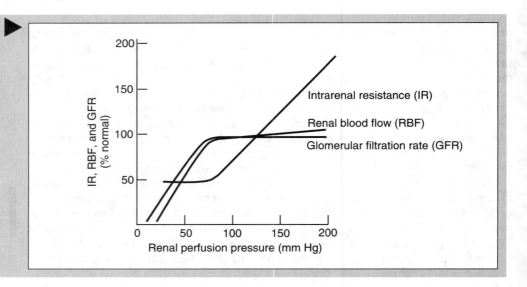

FIGURE 3-4 ▶
Relationships among Glomerular Filtration Rate, Renal Blood Flow, and Calculated Intrarenal Resistance Versus Changes in Renal Perfusion Pressure. Because renal blood flow remains constant as perfusion pressure increases higher than 70 mm Hg, the intrarenal resistance must increase.

The kidney maintains GFR constant over a wide range of perfusion pressures in the absence of external influences.

tion. Because autoregulation can be demonstrated in the isolated kidney as well as in intact subjects, it must be independent of extrinsic factors such as the nervous system or circulating hormones. It also occurs over a wide range of pressures, and many patients with severe hypertension do not have an elevated GFR. Because, as pointed out above, glomerular capillary pressure is the physiologic variable that determines GFR, the obvious conclusion to be drawn is that the glomerular capillary pressure is regulated to maintain a constant GFR even when systemic arterial pressure varies.

The relationship between renal perfusion pressure and both RBF and intrarenal resistance is also shown in Fig. 3-4. When perfusion pressure increases, the intrarenal resistance increases, but RBF is held constant. Recall from Fig. 3-1 that alterations in either afferent or efferent arteriole resistance influence both GFR and blood flow. Two important questions arise: Is the site of the change in intrarenal resistance the afferent or efferent arteriole, and what are the mechanisms involved in the regulation of this resistance during autoregulation?

Afferent Arteriole as Site of Resistance Change

The analogy used in Fig. 3-1 can be used to deduce the site of the resistance change in an autoregulating kidney. When blood pressure increases, the intrarenal resistance also increases. If the increased resistance occurred at the efferent arteriole, blood flow would be held constant because the increased resistance to blood flow would compensate for the increased blood pressure. However, in this case, GFR would be increased because of the increased glomerular capillary pressure upstream from the constriction. In an autoregulating kidney, both GFR and RBF are held constant when blood pressure increases. The obvious conclusion drawn from this analogy is that the change in resistance mediating autoregulation occurs primarily at the afferent arteriole. A change in arterial blood pressure leads to an intrinsic change in afferent arteriolar resistance to maintain glomerular capillary pressure and, therefore, GFR constant. The functional significance of renal autoregulation is to maintain a constant input into the renal tubules. Because the site of autoregulation of GFR is the afferent arteriole, RBF also is regulated. In both normal and pathophysiologic conditions, almost all changes in intrarenal resistance primarily occur at the afferent arteriole. Consequently, both GFR and RBF change in the same relative proportion.

The afferent arteriole is the site of the resistance change that mediates autoregulation.

Mechanisms of Autoregulation

Throughout the years, there have been many theories to explain the mechanisms of renal autoregulation. Two theories that have stood the test of time are now widely accepted. They are the myogenic mechanism theory and the tubuloglomerular feedback theory. These two mechanisms usually act in concert to reinforce each other and do not act exclusively of one another.

Myogenic Mechanism. Reflex changes in afferent arteriole resistance can minimize the effect of changes in arterial pressure on glomerular capillary pressure. It was recognized many years ago that smooth muscle inherently contracts if stretched and relaxes if shortened. Because the afferent arteriole is a smooth-muscle resistance arteriole similar to other systemic resistance vessels, this observation has been applied to the kidney to explain one of the components of autoregulation and has been termed the *myogenic response* (Fig. 3-5). This response is rapid, and it is the first line of defense against rapid changes in blood pressure. An increase in arterial blood pressure results in stretching of the afferent arteriolar wall because of the increased intraluminal pressure. If the arteriole were a rubber tube, the increased pressure would simply be transmitted downstream to increase glomerular capillary pressure and GFR. However, the myogenic mechanism results in a reflex contraction of the arteriole and returns the diameter of the arteriole toward normal. This contraction prevents the total transmission of the increased pressure to the glomerular capillary and minimizes the change in GFR. Conversely, a decrease in arterial pressure results in relaxation. The myogenic mechanism is inherent in the smooth muscle and tends to minimize any change in glomerular capillary pressure in response to changes in arterial blood pressure. In this manner, the glomerular capillary pressure and GFR are maintained at approximately normal values. However, because the myogenic mechanism only *minimizes* the change in glomerular capillary pressure, the tubuloglomerular feedback mechanism is necessary to precisely regulate filtration rate.

Myogenic mechanism
Reflex contraction of smooth muscle in response to increased blood pressure minimizes the downstream increase in the glomerular capillary pressure.

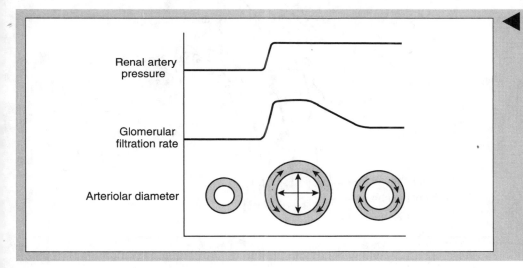

FIGURE 3-5
Myogenic Mechanism for Autoregulation of Glomerular Filtration Rate (GFR). *Increased renal artery pressure transiently increases GFR and arteriolar diameter. Reflex constriction of the arteriole decreases arteriolar diameter and GFR back towards normal.*

Tubuloglomerular Feedback. The human kidney is composed of approximately 1 million individual nephrons. Each of these individual nephrons has a point of contact between the distal nephron and the afferent arteriole of the same nephron. This area of contact and the related structures are collectively known as the *juxtaglomerular apparatus* (Fig. 3-6). An important component of this area is a small number of specialized distal nephron cells called the *macula densa*. The juxtaglomerular apparatus has been shown to play a major role in the regulation of the filtration rate. It has been proposed that changes in delivery or composition of fluid in the distal tubule are sensed by the macula densa cells and, as a result, changes in afferent arteriole resistance are evoked to bring the delivery or composition of the tubular fluid back to normal. A schematic diagram of the anatomic arrangement of the nephron, and the control system for the tubuloglomerular feedback mechanism is shown in Fig. 3-7. Because the major regulator of pressure in the glomerular capillaries is the resistance of the afferent arteriole, and because the juxtaglomerular apparatus is closely associated with the afferent arteriole, the system revolves around changes in *afferent arteriole resistance*. Recall from Chap. 1 that in this type of diagram a *solid line* represents a direct relationship, and a *dashed line* represents an inverse relationship. For the sake of illustration, suppose that blood pressure increases. This would lead to an increase in pressure in the glomerular capillary distal

Each individual nephron has an area of contact between the distal nephron and its own afferent arteriole at the juxtaglomerular apparatus.

FIGURE 3-6 ▶

Schematic Representation of the Juxtaglomerular Apparatus Illustrating the Macula Densa Cells and the Granular Cells in Juxtaposition to the Afferent Arteriole and the Glomerulus.

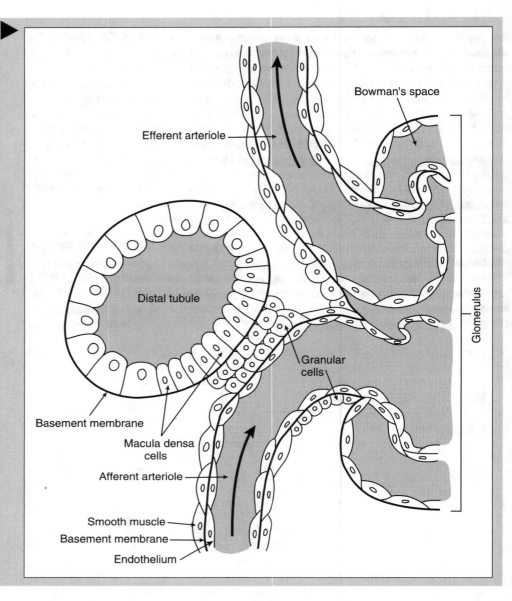

FIGURE 3-7 ▶

Tubuloglomerular Feedback Mechanism for Autoregulation of Glomerular Filtration Rate (GFR). Increased GFR results in increased delivery at the juxtaglomerular apparatus. The JGA causes increased resistance at the afferent arteriole to decrease glomerular capillary pressure. The decreased GC pressure returns GFR and delivery to normal.

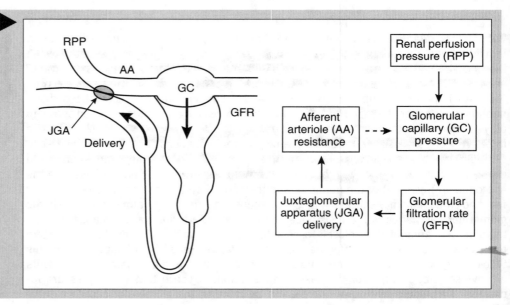

to the afferent arteriole and would increase the GFR. Any increase in GFR would result in increased distal tubular delivery of filtered fluid and solute to the juxtaglomerular apparatus. This increased delivery would be correctly interpreted as an increased GFR, and the resistance of the afferent arteriole would be increased to reduce glomerular capillary pressure and bring GFR back to normal. In the case of an increase in blood pressure, the myogenic mechanism tends to restore capillary pressure to near normal, and the system is fine-tuned by tubuloglomerular feedback. In the case of a decrease in blood pressure, the exact opposite chain of events occurs. Thus, the myogenic mechanism and the tubuloglomerular feedback system act in concert to maintain glomerular capillary pressure at a constant value and to ensure a normal GFR despite the normal daily fluctuations in systemic blood pressure.

Although the tubuloglomerular feedback system is very sensitive to changes in fluid composition at the juxtaglomerular apparatus and is very precise in regulating GFR under normal conditions, several points must be noted. First, the mechanisms by which changes in fluid delivery or composition are transduced to changes in afferent arteriole resistance are unknown and are under intense investigation. For example, it has been proposed that intracellular calcium, adenosine, or adenosine triphosphate (ATP) are involved, but their mechanism of action is not known. In addition, the macula densa cells of the juxtaglomerular apparatus cannot differentiate between true alterations in GFR and alterations in fluid flow rate due to changes in tubular transport proximal to the macula densa. For instance, an increase in GFR or a decrease in proximal tubular reabsorption could give the same change in fluid delivery or composition at the macula densa cells.

> **Tubuloglomerular feedback**
> An increase in delivery of tubular fluid at the juxtaglomerular apparatus results in increased afferent arteriole resistance to decrease glomerular capillary pressure and GFR. The opposite occurs in response to a decreased delivery of tubular fluid.

> The myogenic mechanism and the tubuloglomerular feedback mechanism act in concert to maintain GFR and renal blood flow constant.

EXTRINSIC REGULATION OF GLOMERULAR FILTRATION RATE

As noted above, under normal conditions both GFR and RBF are maintained very constant by the intrinsic myogenic and tubuloglomerular feedback mechanisms existing in the kidney. However, there are many stress conditions in which it is advantageous for the body to decrease both GFR and RBF. Physiologically, the maintenance of appropriate volumes and pressures, particularly the plasma volume and arterial blood pressure, is necessary to adequately perfuse all the organ systems. In times of volume or pressure stress, such as hemorrhage or dehydration, many physiologic influences converge on the kidney to reduce GFR and RBF. Some of these factors are discussed below.

> Homeostatic mechanisms are geared to maintain adequate volumes and pressures of the organism.

Nervous System

The afferent arteriole and the proximal tubule are richly innervated by the sympathetic nervous system. In times of low blood volume, the output of the sympathetic nervous system is greatly increased. A decreased volume status is sensed by the low-pressure receptors in the right heart and pulmonary circulation, whereas a decline in blood pressure is sensed by the high-pressure receptors in the carotid sinus and aortic arch. The net result is a marked increase in sympathetic output to the periphery and a release of catecholamines from the adrenal medulla. The physiologic effects are obvious and advantageous. Sympathetically mediated arteriolar constriction leads to increased peripheral resistance, which tends to maintain the arterial pressure, and the sympathetic effect of increasing the heart rate is a physiologic attempt to maintain cardiac output. Similar to the effects on peripheral vascular arterioles, the increased sympathetic outflow also markedly constricts the afferent arteriole. This constriction decreases glomerular capillary pressure and decreases GFR, preventing further loss of fluid through filtration. It also shunts blood flow to other areas of the body that have a greater need, such as the brain and heart. Major increases in sympathetic outflow also may cause efferent arteriole constriction and further decrease RBF.

Although severely decreased plasma volume is probably the most common pathologic cause of diminished GFR and RBF, a much more physiologic example is that

> The sympathetic nervous system can constrict the afferent arterioles and decrease GFR and RBF.

of short-term severe exercise. The increased autonomic activity that occurs during the onset of severe exercise may reduce GFR and RBF to less than 50% of normal. Whereas long-term strenuous exercise may induce sweating and significant loss of plasma volume, the effect of autonomic nervous system on the kidney can occur almost immediately, well before any loss of volume occurs. In this case, the beneficial effect of the increased renal resistance is to shunt blood to the muscles that need it to function maximally. The shift of blood flow from the kidney to the muscles may have evolved as a survival mechanism for an organism put in a "fight-or-flight" situation.

Angiotensin II

Marked vasoconstriction of the kidney may occur very rapidly during onset of heavy exertion or when fleeing from danger.

Angiotensin II is a potent vasoactive peptide that is intimately involved in both blood pressure regulation and Na+ homeostasis. Although these subjects are discussed at length later, a brief description germane to renal hemodynamics is presented here. The renin–angiotensin system is a cascade of events that begins in the kidney and results in the formation of circulating angiotensin II (Fig. 3-8). Renin is an enzyme that is secreted into the bloodstream by the kidney. The enzyme acts on a circulating globulin previously formed in the liver called renin substrate (sometimes called angiotensinogen). A decapeptide is cleaved from the substrate to form angiotensin I. Angiotensin I is converted to the octapeptide angiotensin II by angiotensin converting enzyme (ACE). Although ACE exists in many tissues, including the kidneys, the major conversion occurs in the lungs. The rate-limiting step in the formation of angiotensin II is the rate of renin secretion by the kidney, because under normal circumstances both renin substrate and ACE exist in excess amounts.

Angiotensin II concentration in the plasma is determined by the rate of renin secretion by the kidney.

FIGURE 3-8 ▶
Schematic Representation of the Renin–Angiotensin System. *The rate-limiting step in the formation of angiotensin II is the rate of renin secretion by the kidney.*

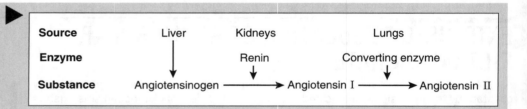

Renin release by the kidney and ultimate formation of angiotensin II is primarily stimulated by baroreceptor-mediated increases in sympathetic nervous activity. Among its other actions, angiotensin II is a potent vasoconstrictor. In times of low volume or pressure, such as would often occur following hemorrhage or dehydration, the addition of another vasoconstrictor represents an additional mechanism to restore pressure toward normal. Thus, the nervous system and the renin–angiotensin system act in concert to prevent the decline in pressure. Constriction of the afferent arteriole decreases glomerular capillary pressure and minimizes the further loss of fluid by glomerular filtration. As with catecholamines, a very high level of circulating angiotensin II not only decreases GFR by afferent arteriolar constriction, but also may constrict the efferent arteriole to further decrease RBF.

Renin release by the kidney and subsequent formation of angiotensin II is stimulated by sympathetic nerves and decreased blood pressure.

The sympathetic nervous system and angiotensin II act together to minimize the decrease in blood pressure in times of excess loss of volume.

There are some pathologic conditions, such as renal artery stenosis, in which the kidney secretes an excess of renin even though blood pressure and volume are normal. In this instance, the underlying stenosis results in a reduction in blood pressure at the afferent arteriole. This decreased pressure is directly perceived by baroreceptors located within the afferent arteriole, and leads to increased renin secretion. The resulting increased generation of angiotensin II leads to an excess constriction of arterioles, including those in the kidney, which may lead to hypertension.

Prostaglandins

Prostaglandins are formed in many tissues from arachidonic acid metabolism, and they often have actions on or near the tissues in which they are formed. Two important prostaglandins formed in the kidney that have actions on the renal arterioles are the vasodilatory prostaglandins, PGE_2 and PGI_2. Although these prostaglandins probably play a minor role in the regulation of normal renal hemodynamics, they may protect the kidneys from excess renal vasoconstriction during times of severe cardiovascular stress such as hemorrhage. The formation of both prostaglandins is stimulated by increased sympathetic nervous system activity and circulating levels of angiotensin II. By stimulating the production of vasodilator prostaglandins, the probability of severe excess constriction by renal sympathetic activity and markedly elevated plasma angiotensin II is obviated (Fig. 3-9). In the example given, a severe decrease in blood pressure would increase sympathetic outflow from the systemic baroreceptors and increase angiotensin II formation through the renin–angiotensin system. Both circumstances could lead to a severe decrease in RBF (renal ischemia). Because one of the major circumstances that potentially can lead to acute renal failure is *complete* renal ischemia, the simultaneous production of the vasodilatory prostaglandins may exert a protective role by preventing severe renal vasoconstriction.

> Prostaglandin synthesis in the kidney is increased by the sympathetic nervous system and angiotensin II.

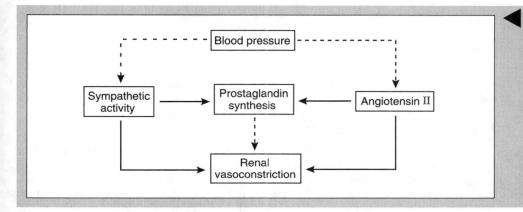

FIGURE 3-9
Interrelationships among the Sympathetic Nervous System, Angiotensin II, and Vasodilatory Prostaglandins. *The severe vasoconstriction caused by the sympathetic nervous system and angiotensin II is modulated by intrarenal synthesis of prostaglandins.*

At times, the blockade of vasodilatory prostaglandins has been found to have deleterious effects on renal function in a clinical setting. For example, in the past, some patients undergoing diagnostic radiology with intravenous contrast medium developed acute renal failure. These patients typically were deprived of fluid overnight, which leads to decreased extracellular volume and increased angiotensin II. In addition, many were given nonsteroidal anti-inflammatory drugs (NSAIDs) for pain or discomfort. A major action of NSAIDs is to prevent the formation of prostaglandins. As a result, the vasoconstrictive influence of increased angiotensin II is unopposed by vasodilatory prostaglandins, and consequently many of these patients developed acute renal failure. It is now common practice to ensure adequate hydration and an intact prostaglandin system before using contrast media in diagnostic studies.

Atrial Natriuretic Peptide (ANP)

ANP, sometimes called atrial natriuretic factor or atriopeptin, is stored primarily in the myocytes of the right atrium from where it is released in response to atrial stretch. It has vasodilatory effects on the peripheral as well as the renal vasculature. The stimulus for release of ANP and the actions of ANP are shown in Fig. 3-10. Increased plasma volume tends to increase pressure in both the high and low pressure side of the circulation, including the right atrium. The increased pressure in the right atrium leads to increased release of ANP. The effect of increased ANP is to return arterial pressure to normal through dilation of the peripheral arterioles. Vasodilatation of the afferent arteriole in the kidney increases glomerular capillary pressure and consequently GFR, which leads to loss of volume through the kidney and returns plasma volume to normal. The net result of the actions of ANP is to return the body to normal pressure and volume and maintain whole body homeostasis. Although it is probable that changes in ANP are not important for the normal regulation of GFR at normal or low plasma volumes, it may be important during times of volume overload and may explain the well-known finding that GFR increases during times of high Na+ intake. In patients with severely decreased GFR caused by chronic renal disease, it is sometimes possible to increase filtration rate by

> ANP is released from the right side of the heart in response to increased right atrial pressure.

> ANP vasodilates systemic and renal arterioles.

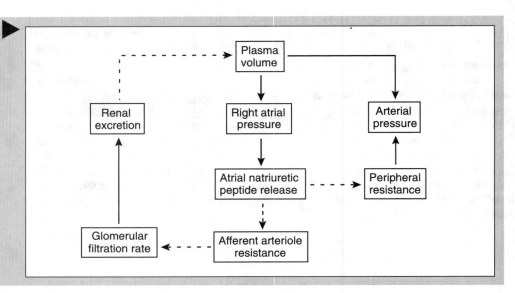

FIGURE 3-10
Hemodynamic Effects of Atrial Natriuretic Peptide. Increased right atrial pressure stimulates the release of atrial natriuretic peptide, which decreases both peripheral and renal vascular resistance.

increasing Na+ intake and extracellular volume. The increased release of ANP may play a role in this mechanism.

Other Vasoactive Substances

There are many vasoactive substances that can affect renal function. Their overall role in the regulation of renal function is under investigation.

Catecholamines, angiotensin II, and ANP have been found to have a role in the regulation of GFR and RBF as well as in the regulation of body fluid volumes and blood pressure. In addition, there are a number of other vasoactive substances that have been found to alter renal hemodynamics (Table 3-1). The overall role of many of these substances in the regulation of renal hemodynamics is equivocal, and the mechanisms regulating their release are under investigation.

TABLE 3-1

Vasoactive Substances

Constriction	Dilatation
Adenosine	Nitric oxide
Angiotensin II	Prostaglandin E_2
Antidiuretic hormone	Acetylcholine
Catecholamines	Atrial natriuretic peptide
Endothelin	Bradykinin

Constriction of the kidney in states of low pressure or volume is a compensatory mechanism that acts with other control systems of the body to minimize the change in pressure or volume.

In light of the fact that the kidney has powerful and precise intrinsic mechanisms to autoregulate GFR and blood flow, what is to be made of the equally powerful extrinsic mechanisms that can also modulate and GFR and RBF? The answer is simple. Under normal conditions the body depends on the kidney to maintain a constant composition and volume of the body fluids, and the kidney maintains homeostasis by filtering and processing the plasma volume many times a day. However, the physiologic control systems of the whole body also are geared to maintain survival. In times of severely low pressure or volume, the kidney may be called upon by the body to minimize the effects of the low pressure or volume. Renal vasoconstriction by extrinsic mechanisms decreases GFR and prevents the further loss of fluid by filtration. Constriction of the renal vasculature also increases peripheral resistance to increase blood pressure and allows the shunting of cardiac output to more needy areas. In this manner, the kidneys act in unison with the other control systems of the body to maintain optimal blood pressure and volume necessary for survival. An example is given in the next section.

SEVERE SWEATING: AN INTEGRATED CARDIORENAL RESPONSE

In the example of severe sweating given in Chap. 1, the intent was to illustrate the fluid shifts that occur with loss of hypotonic fluid from the extracellular space. Here it is used to emphasize the mechanisms by which the body attempts to maintain plasma volume and blood pressure. Mild exertion that results in minimal sweating is a problem that can be corrected by increased fluid intake and physiologic alterations in renal function. However, loss of volume sufficient to reduce plasma volume significantly calls into play additional control systems that tend to prevent further loss of volume and also minimize the decrease in plasma volume and blood pressure (Fig. 3-11).

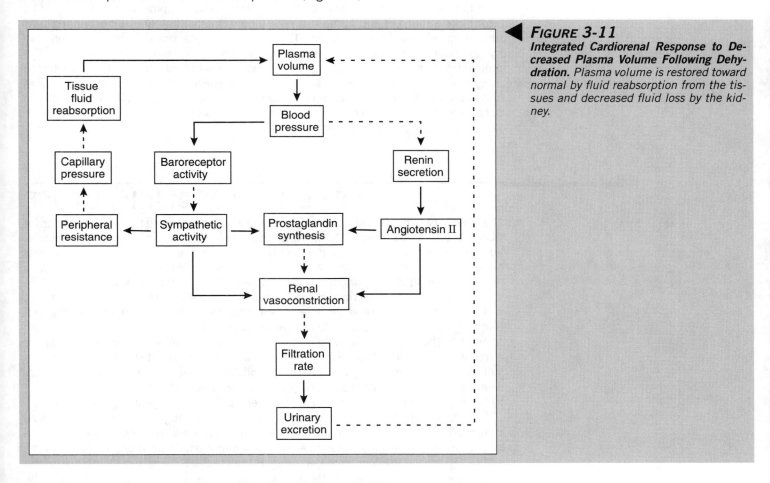

◀ **FIGURE 3-11**
Integrated Cardiorenal Response to Decreased Plasma Volume Following Dehydration. *Plasma volume is restored toward normal by fluid reabsorption from the tissues and decreased fluid loss by the kidney.*

The fundamental disturbance in severe sweating is a decrease in extracellular volume, both from the interstitial space and, more importantly, the plasma volume. The loss of plasma volume tends to decrease blood pressure, and the body responds in several ways. The decreased plasma volume is sensed as a decrease in pressure on the low-pressure side of the cardiovascular system, and the decline in arterial blood pressure is sensed by the high-pressure receptors in the carotid sinus and aortic arch. The decline in blood pressure is minimized by the increased sympathetic outflow, which constricts both renal and peripheral arterioles. The increase in renal resistance decreases GFR to prevent further loss of volume in the urine which tends to maintain the existing plasma volume. In addition, the increased sympathetic outflow and decreased blood pressure stimulate the renal release of renin and the formation of angiotensin II, which further constricts the arterioles. The constriction of the peripheral arterioles leads to decreased capillary pressure downstream from the constriction, whereas the loss of hypotonic fluid as sweat

Fluid lost during sweating comes mainly from the extracellular volume, including the plasma volume.

Increased renal resistance prevents further loss of fluid by decreasing GFR.

Severe sweating leads to decreased systemic capillary pressure and increased plasma colloid osmotic pressure. Both factors promote movement of fluid from the interstitial space into the circulation.

leaves the plasma proteins more concentrated than normal. The decreased capillary pressure and increased plasma colloid osmotic pressure both promote the reabsorption of fluid back into the plasma from the interstitium.

All the physiologic responses to severe sweating are aimed at minimizing the decrease in plasma volume. However, the problem still exists; that is, the plasma volume is still low. The kidneys prevent the further loss of volume, and the peripheral reabsorption of fluid from the interstitium minimizes the decrease in plasma volume. Restoration of the original volume must be accomplished by intake. Only when the lost fluid is replaced does the body return to a state of homeostasis.

It should be pointed out that the described mechanisms also apply to almost any condition in which plasma volume is decreased. For example, donation of a pint of blood results in peripheral constriction and reabsorption of fluid from the interstitial space back into the cardiovascular system to minimize the decrease in plasma volume. However, in this case the decrease in plasma volume is small: approximately 0.5 L out of a total blood volume of 6.0 L. Normal renal hemodynamic function is maintained, and renal autoregulation remains intact. The major role of the kidney in this situation is to increase water and electrolyte reabsorption, which is discussed in later chapters. The protein lost in the donation of the pint of blood is replenished in a matter of days by the liver, and the red blood cells are subsequently replenished by the bone marrow. Severe loss of blood, which may occur during traumatic hemorrhage, brings all the physiologic defense mechanisms into play, including renal vasoconstriction, in an attempt to maintain a functional plasma volume.

RESOLUTION OF CLINICAL CASE

The clinical case presented is not common, and ACE inhibitors are the drugs of choice for many hypertensive patients. The inhibitors have been used in most cases for years with no undue side effects. However, this case does illustrate the relationships between renal autoregulation, blood pressure, and selective renal arteriole resistance. Mr. Smith had a history of hyperlipidemia, which may predispose to atherosclerotic plaques in the peripheral arteries, including the renal arteries. The effect of the occlusion in the renal arteries was to decrease pressure at the afferent arteriole and in the glomerular capillary. The intrinsic myogenic and tubuloglomerular feedback mechanisms were activated in an attempt by the kidney to maintain normal GFR. However, the decreased pressure at the afferent arteriole was also a signal to the kidneys to increase the release of renin to subsequently generate angiotensin II. The physician reasoned correctly that the increased angiotensin II may be responsible for the increased peripheral resistance and hypertension. He prescribed a drug that prevented the formation of angiotensin II.

On follow-up, Mr. Smith's condition was worse. Although his blood pressure was controlled by the ACE inhibitor, the GFR was only about one-sixth of normal, as indicated by the further increased plasma creatinine concentration. In addition, the plasma Na^+ and HCO_3^- concentrations were low, whereas the plasma K^+ was high. The cause of the electrolyte disorder was the greatly decreased GFR, which diminished the ability of the kidney to maintain body fluid homeostasis. Then, why was the GFR low? The answer can be found in the selective constriction of the afferent and efferent arterioles.

On the initial visit, Mr. Smith probably had a severe atherosclerotic constriction of the renal arteries. Despite the elevated systemic blood pressure, the renal artery constriction resulted in a decreased pressure downstream in the afferent arteriole and glomerular capillary. Because the pressure at the juxtaglomerular apparatus remained low, the amount of renin secreted by the afferent arteriole and the amount of angiotensin II generated remained elevated. Because blood pressure had increased, the sympathetic outflow to constrict the afferent arteriole was minimal. The effect of angiotensin II to constrict the afferent arteriole was partially offset by the intrinsic vasodilatory autoregulating mechanisms in the kidney. However, the angiotensin II levels were very high, and the response of the efferent arteriole to high circulating angiotensin II was vasoconstriction. Both vasodilation of the afferent arteriole by intrinsic mechanisms and constriction of the efferent arteriole by angiotensin II tended to maintain glomerular capillary pressure, and GFR was only modestly decreased despite the renal artery stenosis.

When the formation of angiotensin II was prevented by ACE inhibition, the vaso-constriction of the efferent arteriole decreased. Referring to the analogy in Fig. 3-1, it can be seen that a decrease in efferent arteriole resistance leads to a decrease in glomerular capillary pressure and a fall in GFR. As pointed out above, this decreased GFR was responsible for the symptoms found on Mr. Smith's follow-up visit. The initial constriction of the efferent arteriole by angiotensin II in this case was actually appropriate to maintain near-normal glomerular capillary pressure and GFR; a condition that was interrupted by the treatment with the ACE inhibitor.

This case assumes that the renal artery of both kidneys is compromised, which is a rather rare condition. A more common condition is single renal artery stenosis. Whereas many times the contralateral kidney is normal, the major problem with a single renal artery stenosis is one of hypertension caused by the excess angiotensin II produced from the stenotic kidney. Apparent renal function is usually relatively normal. However, hypertension is a serious clinical problem that also can have detrimental effects on the normal kidney. If the stenosis is identified, it often can be repaired surgically.

REVIEW QUESTIONS

Directions: For each of the following questions, choose the **one best** answer.

1. Which of the following physiologic regulators is most important in determining glomerular filtration rate?

    (A) Glomerular capillary hydrostatic pressure

    (B) Bowman's space hydrostatic pressure

    (C) Glomerular capillary colloid osmotic pressure

    (D) Bowman's space colloid osmotic pressure

2. Acetazolamide is a drug commonly given to patients with glaucoma to prevent transport in the eye and reduce intraocular pressure. Acetazolamide also inhibits transport in the proximal tubule of the kidney. If the kidney's tubuloglomerular feedback system is intact following ingestion of acetazolamide, the filtration rate would be expected to

    (A) increase

    (B) decrease

    (C) not change

3. A decrease in efferent arteriolar diameter would be expected to cause which one of the following combinations of changes?

    (A) Increased renal blood flow (RBF) and increased glomerular filtration rate (GFR)

    (B) Increased RBF and decreased GFR

    (C) Decreased RBF and increased GFR

    (D) Decreased RBF and decreased GFR

4. Which one of the following conditions might be associated with increased glomerular filtration rate (GFR)?

    (A) Hypertension

    (B) Edema

    (C) Renal artery stenosis

    (D) Excess Na^+ intake

5. Full restoration of the plasma volume following severe sweating can occur by which one of the following mechanisms?

    (A) Reabsorption of fluid from the interstitial space

    (B) Decrease in water and electrolyte excretion by the kidney

    (C) Increased intake of water and electrolytes

6. An increase in the ultrafiltration coefficient initially results in which one of the following responses?

    (A) Increased glomerular filtration rate (GFR)

    (B) Decreased delivery of tubular fluid to the juxtaglomerular apparatus

    (C) Increased filtration of albumin

    (D) Increased renal blood flow

7. A patient with severe congestive heart failure might be expected to have which one of the following conditions?

    (A) Increased blood pressure caused by increased sympathetic nervous system activity

    (B) Increased plasma creatinine concentration because of decreased glomerular filtration rate (GFR)

    (C) Decreased atrial natriuretic peptide (ANP) release attributed to decreased right atrial pressure

    (D) Increased cardiac output due to increased preload on the heart

8. A patient with a pheochromocytoma might be expected to exhibit symptoms of which one of the following conditions?

    (A) Decreased blood pressure

    (B) Increased sympathetic nervous system activity

    (C) Increased plasma creatinine concentration

    (D) Increased atrial natriuretic peptide (ANP) release

ANSWERS AND EXPLANATIONS

1. **The answer is A.** Hydrostatic pressure in the glomerular capillary is no more important than hydrostatic pressure in Bowman's space or colloid osmotic pressure in the glomerular capillary. They are all equally responsible for fluid movement across the capillary. However, when considering physiologic regulation, the most important is glomerular capillary hydrostatic pressure because it can be intrinsically and extrinsically regulated through changes in afferent arteriolar resistance. Except in times of tubular or ureteral obstruction, Bowman's space pressure is relatively constant. Plasma protein concentration, which is the determinant of colloid osmotic pressure, is regulated by the liver. In normal circumstances, there is no protein in Bowman's space.

2. **The answer is B.** Inhibition of proximal tubule reabsorption should increase delivery to the juxtaglomerular apparatus. The kidney incorrectly perceives this as an increase in filtration rate. The appropriate response is an increase in afferent arteriole resistance, a decrease in glomerular capillary pressure, and a decrease in filtration rate. Although the response of the kidney may seem inappropriate to whole body homeostasis, it is appropriate for the signal perceived by the kidney and, in fact, may be adaptive to minimize excess loss of fluid and electrolytes due to the drug.

3. **The answer is C.** It should be recalled from cardiovascular principles that resistance to blood flow is inversely related to the fourth power of the diameter of the vessel. Or, conversely, conductance is directly proportional to the fourth power of the radius. Thus, a decrease in diameter of either renal arteriole increases resistance and decreases blood flow. In this case, the site of the increased resistance is distal to the glomerular capillary. Identical to the systemic circulation, any increase in resistance leads to increased pressure upstream from the resistance change by impeding outflow of blood. In this case, the upstream vessel is the glomerular capillary. The increased capillary hydrostatic pressure should lead to an increase in GFR accompanied by a decrease in RBF.

4. **The answer is D.** Excess Na^+ intake can lead to increased plasma volume and release of atrial natriuretic peptide (ANP) from the right heart. The effect of ANP is to decrease afferent resistance and increase GFR. It might be anticipated that hypertension would lead to increased glomerular capillary pressure and increased GFR. How-

ever, the kidney autoregulates in the presence of the high blood pressure and maintains a constant GFR. A major cause of edema is decreased plasma protein concentration and loss of fluid into the interstitial space. It might be reasoned that the decreased colloid osmotic pressure in the plasma could lead to increased GFR. However, the source of the edema fluid is the plasma, and plasma volume is decreased. The effect of decreased plasma volume is increased sympathetic nervous system output and increased angiotensin II, both of which constrict the kidney and lead to decreased GFR. Depending on the severity of the renal artery stenosis, GFR may be normal or decreased.

5. **The answer is C.** Reabsorption of fluid from the interstitial space only minimizes the decrease in plasma volume; it does not restore the plasma volume to normal. Similarly, the kidney can prevent only the further loss of water and electrolytes. It cannot manufacture either water or electrolytes, and this point is often overlooked. Full restoration of plasma volume can occur only when the lost volume has been replaced. The importance of intake often is not appreciated, and appropriate monitoring of intake is crucial to the good management of fluid and electrolyte disorders.

6. **The answer is A.** The key to this rather difficult question, "initially results in," indicates a short-term effect without subsequent adjustments. Because the short-term is the concern, the most obvious answer is A. A simple increase in the permeability or area of the glomerular capillary results in increased movement of fluid across the glomerular capillary, although the pressures for filtration do not change. If the kidney can autoregulate, then the glomerular capillary pressure is decreased by the kidney to maintain a normal GFR. The initial increase in GFR increases delivery of tubular fluid to the juxtaglomerular apparatus. This increased delivery is ultimately responsible for the tubuloglomerular feedback increase in afferent arteriole resistance and the restoration of GFR to normal. An increase in the ultrafiltration coefficient alone does not alter filtration of albumin across the glomerular capillary, because it is the negative charge that prevents albumin movement. A simple loss of negative charge increases the filtration of albumin but will not influence the movement of fluid. Initially, blood flow is not changed, but a larger fraction of the blood is filtered. To the extent that afferent arteriole resistance subsequently increases because of autoregulation, then blood flow decreases but GFR is normal.

7. **The answer is B.** Congestive heart failure is characterized by an inability of the left ventricle to pump blood adequately from the pulmonary circulation into the arterial circulation. The failure to provide sufficient cardiac output results in a decrease in systemic blood pressure, which is sensed by the arterial baroreceptors and does indeed result in increased sympathetic nervous system activity. The increased sympathetic activity tends to restore the blood pressure back toward normal. However, it does not increase blood pressure above normal; it only minimizes the decrease. The sustained increase in sympathetic activity increases the constriction of both the peripheral and the renal arterioles and decreases GFR. Because creatinine is removed from the body almost exclusively by filtration and the GFR is decreased, the plasma concentration of creatinine increases. The kidney is perfectly healthy, but the extrinsic influence of the sympathetic nervous system predominates over intrinsic autoregulation. An inability to remove blood from the pulmonary circulation results in a congestion of blood in the pulmonary circulation and is the reason for the term *congestive* heart failure. The increased volume in the low-pressure side of the circulation results in increased pressure in the right side of the heart and should increase— not decrease—the release of ANP. Although an increase in pressure in the pulmonary circulation should increase cardiac output, the problem is an inability of the left side of the heart to pump. Although the increased left atrial pressure may restore cardiac output to near normal, congestion of the pulmonary circulation results in pulmonary edema. In any case, cardiac output only returns to normal and is not increased.

8. **The answer is C.** A pheochromocytoma is a tumor of the adrenal medulla that results in a pathologic excess secretion of catecholamines. Increased catecholamines lead to constriction of the peripheral arterioles. The effect of the increased resistance is an increase in blood pressure. The increased blood pressure is sensed by the arterial baroreceptors, and sympathetic outflow is decreased. The blood pressure is still increased because of the increased circulating catecholamines. The catecholamines also constrict the renal afferent arteriole to decrease glomerular capillary pressure and glomerular filtration rate (GFR). The decreased GFR leads to a retention of creatinine and an increase in plasma creatinine concentration. ANP release may be decreased. The effect of catecholamines on the heart is to increase heart rate and increase contractility. Together, this should increase cardiac output and lower right atrial pressure.

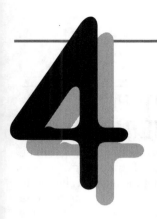

REGULATION OF TUBULAR REABSORPTION

INTRODUCTION OF CLINICAL CASE

A 65-year-old man was admitted to the hospital complaining of chest pain and shortness of breath. He was observed overnight, and a 12-hour urine sample was collected. The 410 mL of urine had an osmolarity of 950 mOsm/L and contained 10 mEq/L of sodium (Na^+). He was diagnosed as having a myocardial infarction with some pulmonary edema, was subsequently treated with digoxin (an oral inotropic agent) and furosemide (a loop diuretic), and was limited to 50 mEq/d of sodium in his diet. In the following 24 hours, he voided 2.8 L of urine, which contained 125 mEq/L of Na^+ and had an osmolarity of 355 mOsm/L. His cardiac function improved, the pulmonary edema resolved, and the diuretic was discontinued. He remained on the digoxin and the low-sodium intake. Several days later 1.4 L of urine was collected over a 24-hour period. The urine osmolarity was 825 mOsm/L, and the urine Na^+ concentration was 30 mEq/L.

ANALYSIS OF RENAL TUBULAR FUNCTION: APPRECIATION OF THE METHODOLOGY

The techniques of in vivo micropuncture and in vitro microperfusion have been essential to increasing our understanding of renal tubular function.

This chapter provides an overview of the unique transport capacities of specific tubule segments. As discussed in previous chapters, the overall renal tubular handling of a given substance can be assessed relatively easily by simply comparing the amount filtered to the amount excreted or, perhaps a little more specifically, by comparing clearance of a substance to the clearance of inulin or creatinine. However, this approach cannot provide any information as to how, for example, the proximal tubule modifies the composition of the glomerular filtrate or as to how much Na^+ is reabsorbed along the collecting tubule system. Two techniques in particular have provided a tremendous amount of information regarding the fundamental function of specific tubule segments, the sites and mechanisms of action of drugs and hormones, and the pathophysiology of renal diseases. These techniques are in vivo micropuncture and in vitro microperfusion (Figs. 4-1 and 4-2).

In Vivo Micropuncture

In vivo micropuncture was originally developed in the 1920s. This technique provides the opportunity to obtain very small (nL) samples of tubular fluid at distinct loci by inserting micropipettes into the tubular lumen. In Fig. 4-1, for example, information concerning the transport capacity of the early proximal tubule can be obtained by comparing the composition of tubular fluid taken from pipette A with the composition of filtered fluid. Similarly, comparing the composition of tubular fluid taken from pipette A with that taken from pipette B provides an estimate of the transport capacity of the loop of Henle. This latter example also illustrates some of the limitations of in vivo micropuncture. For example, tubular fluid can be sampled only from nephron segments that reach the surface of the kidney. Note that pipette A is inserted into the last accessible convolution of the proximal tubule. Beyond this point, tubular fluid must pass through more distal portions of the proximal tubule, as well as thin descending, medullary, and cortical thick ascending limb segments prior to collection at pipette B, which is inserted

FIGURE 4-1 ▶

In Vivo Micropuncture. Glass micropipettes, typically with a tip diameter of 5–10 μm, are inserted into the tubular lumen of nephron segments that are located close to the surface of the kidney. Pipette A is inserted into the last surface-accessible section of the proximal convoluted tubule, and pipette B is inserted into the first surface-accessible section of the distal convoluted tubule. Tubular fluid is withdrawn by applying slight negative pressure to the pipette. Ideally, the rate of withdrawal should be equal to the rate of tubular fluid flow at that point in the nephron.

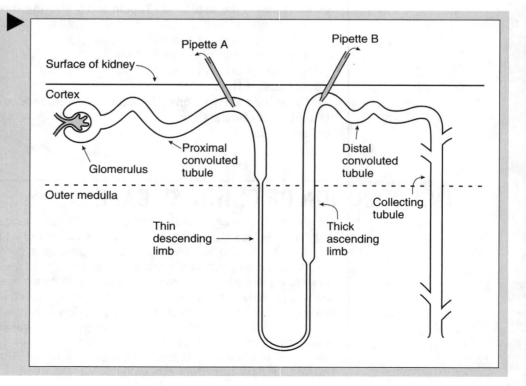

in the first accessible segment of the distal tubule beyond the loop of Henle. Consequently, the change in composition of this fluid is due to the composite effects of all these tubule segments, and micropuncture cannot establish the transport capacity of any one specific segment in this case. Note also that the information derived from these studies can be applied only to superficial (cortical) nephrons. The anatomic location of juxtamedullary nephrons makes micropuncture essentially impossible on this population of nephrons.

In Vitro Microperfusion

More detailed segmental analysis can be accomplished only with in vitro microperfusion. With this technique, specific nephron segments are microdissected from renal tissue and perfused in vitro (see Fig. 4-2). This technique provides an opportunity to precisely control the composition of both the bathing fluid as well as the luminal perfusate and thus affords an opportunity to assess the effects of single agents (e.g., hormones, drugs) on transport function.

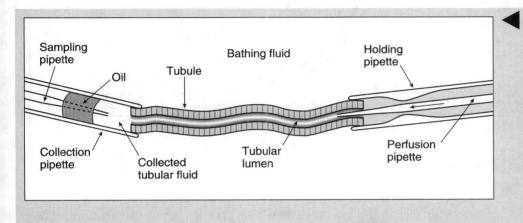

FIGURE 4-2

In Vitro Microperfusion. Freshly microdissected tubular segments, typically 0.5–1.0 mm in length, are transferred to a perfusion chamber. Each end is carefully aspirated into the tip of a glass pipette. On the right, a second small-diameter pipette is inserted into the lumen of the tubule. This pipette is used to perfuse the lumen with a fluid of defined composition. This fluid is collected under oil in the left pipette and withdrawn at regular intervals with a sampling pipette. Fundamentally, the difference in volume and composition between the perfusion fluid and the collected fluid is due to the reabsorptive (or secretory) characteristics of the tubule.

REABSORPTION IN THE PROXIMAL TUBULE

Overall Transport Capacity

Quantitatively, the proximal tubule is the primary site for reabsorption of filtered water and solutes along the renal tubule. Overall, the proximal tubule reabsorbs approximately two-thirds of the glomerular filtrate, although this value can be slightly deceptive. For example, approximately two-thirds of the filtered water and Na^+ are indeed reabsorbed by the time the fluid enters the thin descending limb of the loop of Henle. In absolute terms, this translates to 120 L of water and 17,000 mEq of Na^+ a day. In contrast, a number of other substances, including glucose, amino acids, organic acids, and bicarbonate (HCO_3^-), are essentially completely reabsorbed by the proximal tubule (Fig. 4-3).

Two-thirds of the filtered water (120 L/d) and Na^+ (17,000 mEq/d) are reabsorbed by the proximal tubule.

SODIUM REABSORPTION

Reabsorption of Na^+ occurs along the entire length of the proximal tubule. However, the proximal tubule can be functionally divided into an "early" and "late" section, based on the attendant anions that accompany the Na^+. In the early proximal tubule, Na^+ is primarily reabsorbed along with several different solutes, including glucose, sulphate, P_i, amino acids, and organic acids. Transport of these solutes across the luminal membrane of the early proximal tubule is mediated by a family of Na^+-coupled cotransporters. As described in Chap. 2 for the Na^+–glucose transporter, this reabsorptive process depends on the action of the basolateral membrane Na^+–K^+-ATPase to keep intracellular Na^+

The filtered load of several substances including glucose, amino acids, organic acids, and HCO_3^- is essentially completely reabsorbed by the proximal tubule.

Na^+ reabsorption is coupled to several solutes in the early proximal tubule and is coupled with Cl^- in the late proximal tubule.

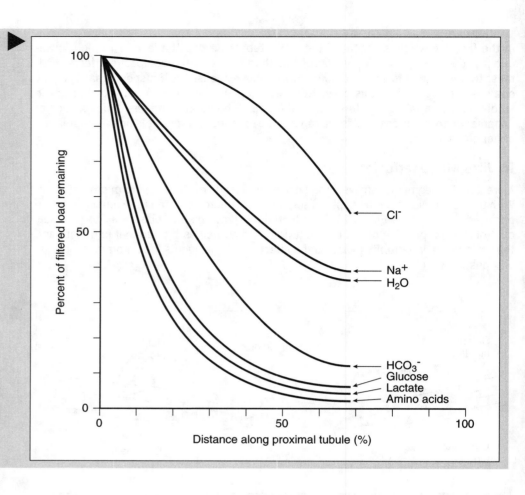

FIGURE 4-3 ▶

Reabsorptive Capacity of the Proximal Tubule. The percentage remaining of the filtered load of several solutes is plotted as a function of the distance along the proximal tubule. Note that data cannot be presented for more than the first 60%–70% of the proximal tubule, since this represents the percentage of the proximal tubule that is accessible to micropuncture.

---

concentration low. In the late proximal tubule, Na+ is preferentially reabsorbed with chloride ion (Cl−). Transport of Na+ across the luminal membrane is now accomplished almost exclusively via a Na+–H+-exchanger. By this point, the reabsorption of water that occurred in the early proximal tubule has generated a tubular fluid with a relatively high Cl− concentration. Consequently, Cl− crosses the luminal membrane down a favorable concentration gradient via a Cl−–organic anion antiporter. This favorable electrochemical gradient also promotes paracellular (between cell) transport of Cl− (Fig. 4-4).

ATYPICAL REABSORPTIVE PROCESSES

The reabsorption of two additional solutes also deserves further consideration. As alluded to earlier, HCO_3^- is avidly reabsorbed in the proximal tubule. However, the reabsorptive mechanism for HCO_3^- is very different from that of many other solutes (Fig. 4-5). In fact, the filtered HCO_3^- is not reabsorbed at all in the traditional sense. The entire process depends on the operation of a Na+–H+ exchanger on the luminal membrane. Within the proximal tubule cell, the enzyme carbonic anhydrase facilitates the conversion of carbon dioxide (CO_2) and water (H_2O) to hydrogen ion (H+) and HCO_3^-. The H+ is secreted into the tubular lumen, where it combines with a filtered HCO_3^- to ultimately form CO_2 and H_2O, again under the influence of carbonic anhydrase that is also located on the luminal membrane. CO_2 and H_2O are then reabsorbed. This "conversion" process has thus prevented a filtered HCO_3^- from being excreted. For each H+ ion that is secreted, and thus for each filtered HCO_3^- ion that is converted, one HCO_3^- ion generated within the proximal tubule cell is transported across the basolateral membrane into the peritubular capillaries; that is, HCO_3^- has effectively been reabsorbed.

The second issue relates to protein. In previous chapters, it was emphasized that the permeability characteristics of the glomerular capillaries prevent plasma proteins from being filtered. In fact, this is not completely correct. Low-molecular-weight proteins can pass through this filtration barrier. However, little if any protein is excreted because these filtered proteins are reabsorbed in the proximal tubule. Similar to HCO_3^-, the reabsorp-

> *The mechanism for the reabsorption of HCO_3^- is indirect and is dependent on H+ secretion into the tubular lumen.*

> *Low-molecular-weight proteins can be filtered, but reabsorption in the proximal tubule prevents them from being excreted.*

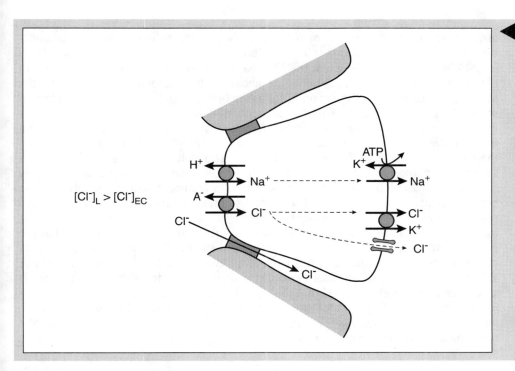

FIGURE 4-4
Cl^- Reabsorption in the Late Proximal Tubule. Cl^- is reabsorbed both transcellularly as well as paracellularly. For the transcellular route, Cl^- and Na^+ enter the cell across the luminal membrane via Cl^--anion and Na^+-H^+-antiporters respectively. Several anions may be used including formate and oxalate. Cl^- that enters the cell exits across the basolateral membrane via a K^+-Cl^--symporter and via a Cl^--selective channel. The high luminal Cl^- concentration in the late proximal tubule also provides an adequate driving force for passive diffusion across the tight junctions. [ ] represents the concentration of Cl^- in the tubular lumen (L) or extracellular fluid (EC).

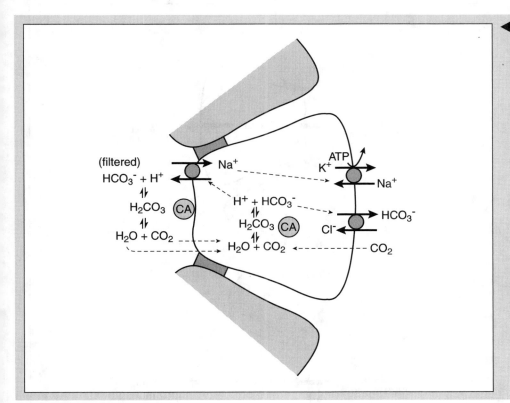

FIGURE 4-5
Reabsorption of HCO_3^- in the Proximal Tubule. Intracellularly, carbonic anhydrase (CA) catalyzes a reaction whereby CO_2 and H_2O initially combine to form carbonic acid, which then dissociates into H^+ and HCO_3^-. The HCO_3^- is transported out of the cell across the basolateral membrane via a HCO_3^--Cl^--antiporter. The H^+ is secreted into the tubular lumen via a Na^+-H^+-antiporter where it reacts with a filtered HCO_3^- molecule. Again under the influence of luminal membrane carbonic anhydrase, the carbonic acid product dissociates into H_2O and CO_2, which can be passively reabsorbed by the renal tubule. The net effect is that for each H^+ secreted into the lumen, one luminal HCO_3^- is "converted" and thus not excreted, and one newly created HCO_3^- is added to the extracellular fluid.

tive process is somewhat atypical. In this case, the filtered proteins are partially digested by proteolytic enzymes located on the luminal membrane prior to cellular uptake by endocytosis. Once inside the cell, the proteins are further broken down into their constituent amino acids and ultimately returned to the bloodstream.

WATER REABSORPTION

As in other nephron segments, the reabsorption of water in the proximal tubule depends on the presence of an osmotic gradient. At first glance, however, it appears that such an osmotic pressure gradient does not exist across the proximal tubule, because micropuncture analysis has established that the osmolarity of the tubular fluid remains essentially isotonic along the entire length of the proximal tubule and, thus, is in equilibrium with the surrounding cortical interstitium. The answer to this apparent paradox is that the reabsorption of water in the proximal tubule is tightly coupled to the reabsorption of solute. Fig. 4-6 provides a somewhat conceptual idea of the sequence of events that facilitates this process. Basically, if solute reabsorption is considered to occur first, then the net movement of solute across the cell generates a slightly hypertonic environment on the basolateral aspect of the cell, whereas removal of solute from the lumen creates a slightly hypotonic tubular fluid. Although the net osmotic gradient may be relatively small (3–4 mOsm/kg), it is more than sufficient to promote water reabsorption in the proximal tubule. Directionally, this water reabsorption occurs both transcellularly and paracellularly, which reflects the fact that the cell membranes, as well as the intervening tight junctions, are extremely water permeable. Therefore, it is not surprising that the proximal tubule is often described as a "leaky epithelium." One additional issue should be appreciated. To this point, it has been emphasized that the primary movement of solute across the proximal tubule provides a driving force for water reabsorption. It should be recognized, however, that the flux of water, particularly via the paracellular route, provides a driving force for the reabsorption of some solutes, including potassium ion (K^+) and calcium ion (Ca^{2+}). Quite simply, this is due to solvent drag, whereby the high rate of water flux simply carries dissolved solutes along with it.

FIGURE 4-6 ▶

Water Reabsorption in the Proximal Tubule. *Step 1: Primary transport of solute across the luminal membrane slightly decreases tubular fluid (TF) osmolarity, and subsequent transport of this solute across the basolateral membrane slightly increases the osmolarity of the extracellular (EC) fluid. Step 2: Since the proximal tubule is a very leaky epithelium, this small osmotic gradient is sufficient to drive reabsorption of a large volume of H_2O both transcellularly and paracellularly.*

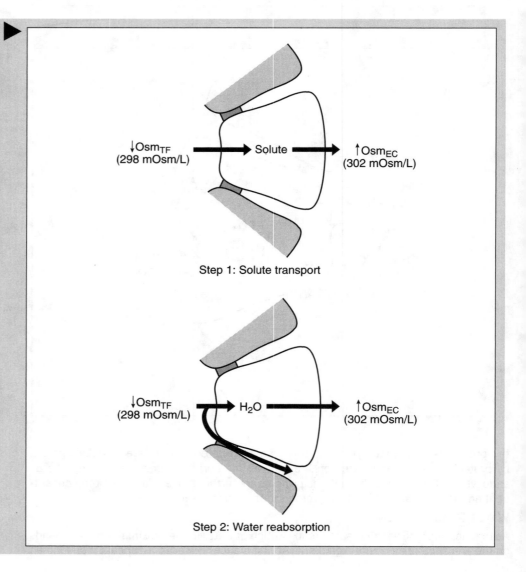

$\downarrow Osm_{TF}$
(298 mOsm/L) → Solute → $\uparrow Osm_{EC}$
(302 mOsm/L)

Step 1: Solute transport

$\downarrow Osm_{TF}$
(298 mOsm/L) → H_2O → $\uparrow Osm_{EC}$
(302 mOsm/L)

Step 2: Water reabsorption

During the past few years, it has become apparent that the water permeability of the luminal and basolateral cell membranes is enhanced by specific water channels, now referred to as aquaporins. As will become apparent as other nephron segments are considered, molecular analysis has established that at least four such aquaporins are expressed within renal epithelial cells. In the proximal tubule, both the luminal and basolateral membranes contain aquaporin-1 (AQP-1) channels.

> *The water permeability of the proximal tubule is enhanced by the presence of specific water channels known as aquaporins.*

Regulation of Proximal Tubule Reabsorption

Despite the magnitude of proximal tubule reabsorption, there are surprisingly few circulating factors that regulate this process. Those that have been identified are listed in Table 4-1 and include extrinsic factors, such as angiotensin II and renal sympathetic nerves, which can increase Na+ reabsorption; atrial natriuretic factor and parathyroid hormone (PTH) are inhibitory. Additionally, several intrarenally synthesized factors also can affect reabsorption. For example, dopamine is recognized as a potent inhibitor of proximal tubule reabsorption.

TABLE 4-1
Potential Modulators of Fluid Reabsorption in the Proximal Tubule

Agonist	Effect on Fluid Reabsorption
Angiotensin II	↑
Catecholamines	↑
Parathyroid hormone	↓
Atrial natriuretic peptide	↓
Dopamine	↓

Note. The effect of each factor is represented as either increasing (↑) or decreasing (↓) fluid reabsorption in the proximal tubule. Most of the available evidence is derived from either in vivo micropuncture or in vitro microperfusion studies.

PROXIMAL TUBULE DIURETICS

The administration of diuretics typically increases both solute and water excretion. Mechanistically, most diuretics inhibit Na+ reabsorption, although the means by which this is accomplished varies considerably. Proximal tubule reabsorption can be modulated by two classes of diuretics: simple osmotic diuretics (e.g., the sugar mannitol) and carbonic anhydrase inhibitors (e.g., acetazolamide). Osmotic diuretics fundamentally upset the very delicate osmotic balance that exists between proximal tubular fluid and the interstitium. Fluid reabsorption in the proximal tubule depends on the maintenance of a small but effective osmotic gradient across the cell. Mechanistically, it is proposed that the initial reabsorption of Na+ causes a slight increase in interstitial osmolarity and a concomitant slight decrease in tubular fluid osmolarity. Given the high water permeability of the proximal tubule, this gradient is sufficient to drive water reabsorption (see Fig. 4-6). Because of solvent drag, a significant amount of solute is also carried along with the water that is reabsorbed paracellularly. Consider, then, the impact of having a relatively high concentration of a freely filterable but poorly reabsorbed solute such as mannitol present in the tubular fluid. As mannitol travels down the proximal tubule, its concentration increases as a result of water reabsorption until it reaches a point where the favorable osmotic gradient no longer exists. As a result, both water reabsorption and the reabsorption of solute that normally occurs by solvent drag are reduced. This mannitol example is clearly an experimental scenario because the sugar must be infused to attain the high tubular fluid concentrations required. However, a very similar situation occurs clinically in patients with diabetes mellitus, in whom the lack of or ineffectiveness of circulating insulin results in a dramatic increase in plasma glucose concentration. As described in Chap. 2, the marked increase in the filtered load of glucose exceeds the transport maximum. Consequently, a considerable amount of glucose is retained within the tubular lumen and acts as an osmotic diuretic. Therefore, one consequence of diabetes mellitus is volume depletion and dehydration as a result of reduced proximal tubule reabsorption of sodium chloride (NaCl) and water.

> *Diuretics increase solute and water excretion and typically act by inhibiting Na+ reabsorption.*

Osmotic diuretics and carbonic anhydrase inhibitors such as acetazolamide inhibit fluid reabsorption in the proximal tubule.

The carbonic anhydrase inhibitors act in a very different manner. The somewhat indirect process of HCO_3^- reabsorption in the proximal tubule depends on the activity of the enzyme carbonic anhydrase and on the ability to secrete H^+ ions into the tubular lumen (see Fig. 4-5). If this enzyme is inhibited, the intracellular generation of H^+ and HCO_3^- ions is reduced. As a result, Na^+ reabsorption is decreased because the luminal membrane Na^+–H^+-antiporter no longer operates optimally, and, thus, filtered HCO_3^- is not converted and effectively reabsorbed. Overall, this drop in solute reabsorption again negatively affects the osmotic balance across the proximal tubule, and water reabsorption is also reduced. However, these diuretics are not in common use because a major side effect is that the failure to reabsorb HCO_3^- almost certainly leads to an inappropriate increase in HCO_3^- excretion and thus a state of systemic acidosis.

STARLING FORCES AND PROXIMAL TUBULE REABSORPTION

The reabsorption of fluid by the proximal tubule is governed by Starling forces.

Despite the relative paucity of extrinsic factors that can alter fluid reabsorption in the proximal tubule, there is considerable intrinsic ability to modulate this reabsorptive process. In Chap. 3, the central role that Starling forces play in glomerular filtration was stressed. These same forces also play a major role in proximal tubule reabsorption. As illustrated in Fig. 4-7, reabsorption is really a two-phase process. Phase 1, which was just discussed, involves the movement of solutes and water from the tubular lumen through the cell and into the interstitium. Phase 2 involves the movement of these substances from the interstitium into the peritubular capillary. It is this latter process that is governed by Starling forces.

Low hydrostatic pressure and high oncotic pressure in the peritubular capillaries promote fluid reabsorption by the proximal tubule.

As with the systemic circulation, but in contrast to the glomerulus, four components need to be taken into consideration, namely interstitial (IN) and peritubular capillary (PC) hydrostatic (P) and colloid osmotic (π) pressures. Fundamentally, the process of glomerular filtration that occurs upstream of the peritubular capillaries creates a balance of Starling forces that favors net reabsorption. First, P_{PC} (a force that opposes

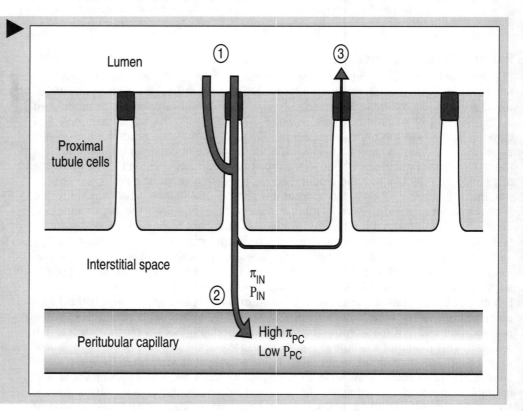

FIGURE 4-7

Role of Starling Forces in Proximal Tubule Fluid Reabsorption. *Fluid transported across and between the proximal tubule cells (1) will either be taken up by the peritubular capillaries (2) or will reflux back into the tubular lumen across the intercellular tight junctions (3). Typically, the favorable balance of Starling forces favors uptake of most of this fluid into the peritubular capillaries.*

reabsorption) is extremely low due to the upstream location of the two major resistance points of the renal circulation (i.e., the afferent and efferent arterioles). Second, π_{PC} (which promotes reabsorption) is high because approximately 20% of the plasma that enters the glomerulus is filtered, thereby increasing the nonfiltered protein concentration in the downstream peritubular capillaries. If P_{PC} increases or if π_{PC} decreases, proximal tubular reabsorption decreases, but the reason for the decrease may not be immediately obvious. One fact not considered earlier is that even under normal circumstances, the total volume of tubular fluid that is transported across the proximal tubular cells is not taken up by the peritubular capillaries. In fact, a relatively small percentage of this fluid fluxes back into the tubular lumen across the tight junctions. At this point, if the driving force for peritubular capillary uptake of fluid is decreased by the change in Starling forces described above, net reabsorption decreases primarily because a greater percentage of fluid transported across the tubular cells refluxes back into the tubular lumen.

GLOMERULOTUBULAR BALANCE

This coupling between resistance at the glomerulus and proximal tubular reabsorption helps to explain the concept of glomerulotubular balance (GT balance). The proximal tubule typically reabsorbs approximately 67% of the filtered load of Na^+ and water. What happens if there is an acute increase in glomerular filtration rate (GFR) and thus the filtered load? In fact, proximal tubular reabsorption also increases such that approximately 67% of this new filtered load is reabsorbed. This ability to alter reabsorptive capacity in response to changes in GFR is referred to as GT balance. This is one mechanism that prevents inappropriate losses of Na^+ and water in the urine that can occur as a result of abrupt increases in GFR.

An Extreme but Illustrative Example. Under normal circumstances, the filtered load of Na^+ is 17.5 mEq/min (125 mL/min $\times$ 0.14 mEq/mL). Of this filtered load, 11.7 mEq/min (67%) is reabsorbed by the proximal tubule. If GFR increases by 5% to 131 mL/min, then the filtered load of Na^+ increases to 18.4 mEq/mL. If the proximal tubule reabsorbed a constant *amount* of the filtered load (11.7 mEq/min), this increase in GFR could potentially result in an additional 0.9 mEq/min of Na^+ (18.4-17.5 mEq) being lost in the urine. However, the proximal tubule will in fact reabsorb 67% of this new filtered load (12.3 mEq/min). Consequently, only an additional 0.3 mEq/min of Na^+ will exit the proximal tubule as a result of this increase in GFR. As we shall see in later sections, more distal nephron segments also have the ability to alter their reabsorptive capacity for Na^+. Consequently most of this additional Na^+ that is delivered distally will also be reabsorbed. Overall therefore, these compensatory mechanisms will prevent a large increase in Na^+ excretion occurring as a result of an acute increase in GFR.

How, then, can the reabsorptive capacity of the proximal tubule be altered to maintain GT balance? At least two mechanisms are thought to be involved. The first mechanism concerns the fact that Na^+ reabsorption in the proximal tubule occurs predominantly via a family of cotransport proteins. Consequently, when GFR increases, the filtered load of glucose and amino acids increases. As we discussed in Chap. 2, the T_m for glucose normally exceeds the filtered load. Consequently, the increase in the filtered load of glucose can be reabsorbed, and because the transport of glucose and Na^+ is coupled, this also results in an increase in Na^+ reabsorption. This increased solute reabsorption also increases water reabsorption. The second mechanism involves the changes in peritubular capillary hydrostatic pressure (P_{PC}) and peritubular capillary oncotic pressure (π_{PC}) that can occur as a result of the change in GFR. For example, as discussed in Chap. 3, an increase in efferent arteriolar resistance increases GFR. Assuming a constant renal plasma flow, this increase in GFR results in an increase in π_{PC} because of the accentuated concentration of plasma proteins along the glomerular capillaries. At the same time, the increased resistance at the efferent arteriole causes a further decrease in P_{PC}. As a result of this shift in Starling forces, net proximal tubule reabsorption will increase (see Fig. 4-8).

> *The ability of the proximal tubule to reabsorb a constant percentage of the filtered load of water and solute is referred to as glomerulotubular (GT) balance.*

FIGURE 4-8 ▶

Impact of Variable Efferent Arteriolar Resistance on Proximal Tubule Fluid Reabsorption.

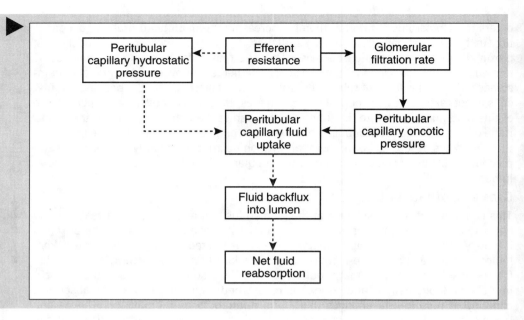

REABSORPTION IN THE LOOP OF HENLE

Hypertonic Medullary Interstitium

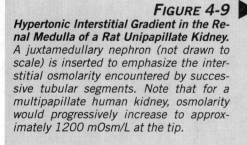

The osmolarity of the medullary interstitium gradually increases from isotonicity at the junction with the cortex to 1200–1400 mOsm/L at the tip of the papilla, as a result of the selective deposition of NaCl and urea.

Before considering the specific transport characteristics of each loop segment, it is important to appreciate the fact that in contrast to the isotonic interstitium of the cortex, the osmolarity of the renal medullary interstitium progressively increases from isotonicity at the corticomedullary junction to markedly hypertonic at the tip of the papilla. In humans, osmolarity can reach 1200–1400 mOsm/L while in the rat, papillary osmolarity approaches 3000 mOsm/L (Fig. 4-9). Several facts deserve special emphasis. First, this hypertonic environment results from the selective deposition of both NaCl and urea within the interstitial space, and as shall be seen in later sections of this chapter and Chap. 5, it is essential to the process of urine concentration. Second, the generation and maintenance of this hypertonic environment depends on the unique permeability characteristics of loop segments, as well as the collecting tubule system.

FIGURE 4-9 ▶

Hypertonic Interstitial Gradient in the Renal Medulla of a Rat Unipapillate Kidney.
A juxtamedullary nephron (not drawn to scale) is inserted to emphasize the interstitial osmolarity encountered by successive tubular segments. Note that for a multipapillate human kidney, osmolarity would progressively increase to approximately 1200 mOsm/L at the tip.

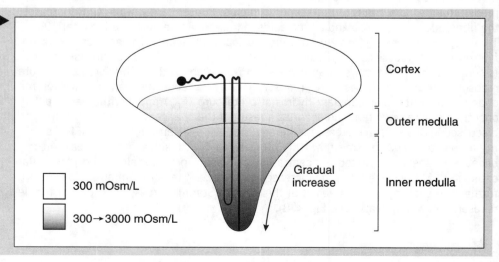

Finally, it should also be appreciated that this very unique environment creates a number of challenges for cells within the medulla. For example, as will be discussed later, the interstitial osmolarity fluctuates, and therefore cells must be capable of adjusting volume to compensate for the osmotic shifts of water that inevitably occur (see Chap. 1). Additionally, cells located within the medulla also must be capable of withstanding high intracellular concentrations of membrane-permeable urea, which is typically considered to be a protein perturbant. Current evidence suggests that within the medulla, several unique solutes, including glycerophosphorylcholine, betaine, sorbitol, and inositol may contribute to both long-term volume regulation and to protein stabilization.

Thin Descending Limb of the Loop of Henle

The permeability characteristics of the thin descending limb are very different from those of the proximal tubule. The thin limb is capable of water reabsorption, but it is not able to reabsorb NaCl. This results from the presence of water channels (AQP-1) in both the luminal and basolateral membrane, while Na⁺-selective transport proteins or channels are absent from the luminal membrane. Consequently, isotonic fluid entering the descending limb from the proximal tubule becomes progressively more concentrated as it descends through a medullary environment of increasing interstitial osmolarity, which provides the driving force for water reabsorption.

The extent to which the tubular fluid is concentrated is basically dictated by the length of the limb segment (Fig. 4-10). Tubular fluid at the end of the descending limb of

> The thin descending limb reabsorbs water but has no capacity to reabsorb NaCl.

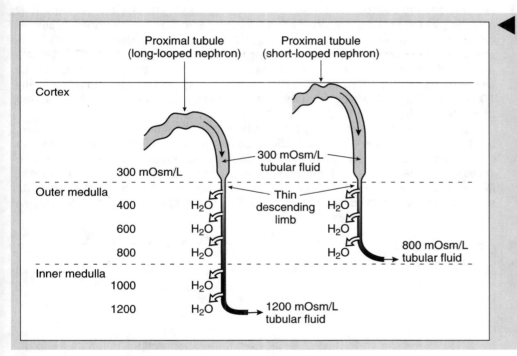

◀ **FIGURE 4-10**
Selective Reabsorption of Water by the Thin Descending Limb of the Loop of Henle. *Selective reabsorption leads to the generation of a hypertonic tubular fluid that is delivered to the ascending limb. Note that the extent to which tubular fluid is concentrated is dependent on the length of the loop and thus the degree to which it traverses the hypertonic medulla. The figure compares a cortical (short-looped) nephron with a juxtamedullary (long-looped) nephron, which descends essentially to the tip of the papilla.*

a human long-looped nephron, for example, should be equal to the osmolarity of the papillary tip interstitium (1200–1400 mOsm/L). Back-calculating, this translates to the reabsorption of a considerable volume of water. Recall that of the 180 L of water that is filtered each day, approximately two-thirds are reabsorbed in the proximal tubule. Consequently, 60 L of isotonic fluid enters the descending limbs daily. If all nephrons were of the long-looped variety, approximately 40 L of water would be reabsorbed to raise the osmolarity of the tubular fluid to 1200 mOsm/L. In the human kidney, in which short-loop nephrons predominate, the descending limbs overall are responsible for the reabsorption of approximately 20 L of water a day. One question frequently asked when considering this mechanism is why the hypertonic interstitial gradient is not diluted out as a result of the reabsorption of so much water by the thin descending limb? The answer is that this water (just as in the cortex) must be immediately taken up by peritubular capillaries. In this case, the medullary peritubular capillaries are the specialized vasa recta, which are discussed in more detail later in the chapter.

To date, little evidence suggests that this reabsorptive process in the thin descending limb is under hormonal control. The extent to which the tubular fluid is concentrated is dictated by the prevailing interstitial osmolarity and the length of any one descending limb.

Ascending Limb of the Loop of Henle

The permeability characteristics of the ascending limb are essentially opposite to those of the descending limb. In this segment, NaCl is in fact very avidly reabsorbed, while the capacity to reabsorb water is essentially zero. In this regard, the ascending limb is quite unique in being one of the few nephron segments that does not express an aquaporin isoform. Overall, the ascending limb is responsible for the reabsorption of approximately 20–25% of the filtered load of NaCl. The driving force for this reabsorptive process is the Na^+-K^+-ATPase located on the basolateral membrane (Fig. 4-11). Transport across the luminal membrane is mediated predominantly by a $Na^+-K^+-2\ Cl^-$-cotransporter. It is this cotransporter that is inhibited by the "loop diuretics" such as furosemide and bumetanide, resulting in inhibition of NaCl reabsorption (see Chap. 2). Most of the K^+ that enters the cell via this cotransporter is not reabsorbed. Rather, it refluxes back into the tubular lumen via luminal membrane K^+ channels. This reflux serves two purposes. First, it ensures an adequate supply of K^+ for the cotransporter, which, if lacking any one ion, would fail to transport all three. Second, this reflux generates a net lumen-positive potential, which provides the driving force for the paracellular reabsorption of several cations including Na^+, K^+, Ca^{2+} and magnesium ion (Mg^{2+}). The net result of this selective solute reabsorption in the ascending limb is that the hypertonic fluid that enters from the descending limb becomes progressively more dilute, to the extent that at the end of the cortical thick ascending limb, tubular fluid is markedly hypotonic (typically 100–120 mOsm/L). Perhaps not surprisingly the thick ascending limb is often referred to as the "diluting segment" of the nephron (Fig. 4-12).

Up to this point, the ascending limb has been considered a homogeneous structure, but this is not the case. First, the thick ascending limb is divided into medullary and cortical segments. In vitro microperfusion studies have revealed that there are differences in both the fundamental transport characteristics and in the regulation of transport in these two segments. For the purposes of this text, however, these differences are quite subtle, and thus we can consider them as one. The long-looped nephrons possess both a

> The thick ascending limb is known as the "diluting segment" of the nephron, since selective reabsorption of NaCl without concomitant water reabsorption generates a hypotonic tubular fluid.

FIGURE 4-11 ▶
NaCl Reabsorption by the Thick Ascending Limb of the Loop of Henle. *Most of the K^+ that enters the cell on the $Na^+-K^+-2Cl^-$-cotransporter refluxes back into the lumen via K^+-selective channels and is thought to serve two purposes. First, this reflux ensures a sufficient luminal concentration of K^+ for optimal function of the cotransporter. Second, the resulting net positive potential in the lumen facilitates paracellular reabsorption of several cations.*

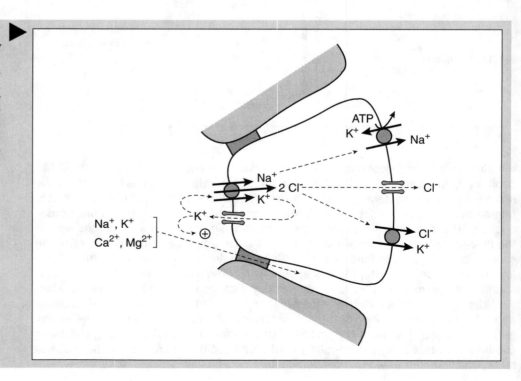

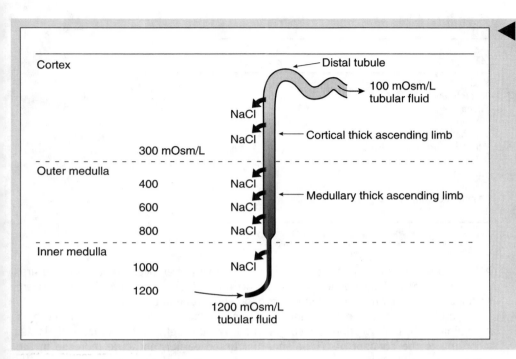

FIGURE 4-12
Selective Reabsorption of NaCl by the Ascending Limb of the Loop of Henle. Selective reabsorption leads to the generation of a hypotonic tubular fluid delivered to the distal tubule.

thick ascending and a thin ascending limb segment, the latter being located predominantly within the inner medulla (see Chap. 2). The thin ascending limb must also reabsorb NaCl; however, the underlying cellular mechanism of reabsorption must be very different from that in the thick limb, since available data suggest that the thin limb cannot sustain active transport to the same extent as the thick segment. In fact, a favorable electrochemical gradient exists to sustain relatively passive reabsorption of NaCl out of the thin ascending limb. This passive model, although not universally accepted, can be explained as follows. If we compare the *osmolarity* of tubular fluid at the very beginning of a long-looped thin ascending limb to that of the interstitium at the same level, they are very similar. However, the *composition* of these two solutions is very different. The hypertonic medullary interstitium results from the selective deposition of both NaCl and urea. Within the inner medulla, these solutes exist in a roughly 1:1 osmolar ratio. In contrast, given the avid reabsorption of many solutes by the proximal tubule, the tubular fluid that flows through the loop of Henle consists predominantly of NaCl. Consequently, although isosmotic, the concentration of NaCl is actually higher in the tubular fluid than in the surrounding interstitium. This concentration gradient facilitates passive reabsorption of NaCl from lumen to interstitium. As an example, a 1000 mOsm/L interstitium consists of 500 mM urea and 250 mM NaCl (remember from Chap. 1 that NaCl dissociates into two particles, thus 250 mM NaCl = 500 mOsm/L). In contrast, at a corresponding level, 1000 mOsm/L tubular fluid could contain 300–400 mM NaCl. As a result, there is a significant chemical (concentration) gradient to support the passive reabsorption of NaCl.

> Reabsorption of NaCl is active in the thick ascending limb and passive in the thin ascending limb.

Regulation of Sodium Chloride Reabsorption in the Thick Ascending Limb

The reabsorption of NaCl in the thick ascending limb is essential to the process that creates the hypertonic medullary interstitium. In sheer magnitude, reabsorption of 25% of the filtered load of NaCl translates to 6000 mEq/d. There is increasing evidence to suggest that this critical reabsorptive process is under significant endocrine control. A number of studies in the 1970s and 1980s supported the concept that arginine vasopressin stimulated NaCl reabsorption in this segment. However, the concensus is now that this is a species-specific response and that it probably does not occur in the human kidney. Table 4-2 provides a listing of other putative modulators of NaCl reabsorption in the ascending limb. The inhibitory effects of a number of these agents, such as atrial natriuretic peptide

TABLE 4-2 ▶

Potential Modulators of NaCl Reabsorption in the Thick Ascending Limb

Note. The effect of each factor is represented as either increasing (↑) or decreasing (↓) NaCl reabsorption in the thick ascending limb of the loop of Henle. Most of the available evidence is derived from either in vivo micropuncture or in vitro microperfusion studies. The general term of adrenal steroids is included in the table, since there are conflicting data regarding the role of either mineralo- or glucocorticoids in this stimulatory response.

Agonist	Effect on NaCl Reabsorption
Arginine vasopressin	↑
Isoproterenol	↑
Glucagon	↑
Insulin	↑
Adrenal steroids	↑
Atrial natriuretic peptide	↓
Adenosine	↓
Bradykinin	↓
Dopamine	↓
Platelet-activating factor	↓
Urodilatin	↓

(ANP), bradykinin and dopamine, are all consistent with their overall natriuretic nature. Additionally, some of these agents appear to have multiple sites of action, since many were included in an earlier listing of modulators of proximal tubular transport.

In addition to putative endocrine/paracrine regulators of reabsorption in the thick ascending limb, reabsorption is also governed by fluid delivery to the loop of Henle. According to the concept of GT balance discussed earlier, an acute increase in the filtered load of NaCl will result in an increase in proximal tubular reabsorption. We alluded to the fact that most of the additional filtered NaCl that is not reabsorbed by the proximal tubule will be reabsorbed by more distal nephron segments. The thick ascending limb is one such segment. In this scenario, an increased delivery of NaCl to the thick ascending limb results in increased reabsorption. The mechanism underlying this delivery dependence is unknown.

There are a number of conditions that result in impaired function of the thick ascending limb. For example, one of the many consequences of adrenal insufficiency is a reduced capacity to reabsorb NaCl from this segment of the nephron, which adversely affects the ability both to concentrate and dilute the urine. In this situation, it is assumed that glucocorticoid and/or mineralocorticoid hormones exert a permissive effect on transport. A more specific pathophysiologic condition that is due almost exclusively to impaired transport in the thick ascending limb is Bartter's syndrome. This condition is caused by a mutation in the luminal membrane $Na^+-K^+-2Cl^-$-cotransporter, and results in volume depletion, renal salt wasting, hyperreninemic hyperaldosteronism, hypercalciuria, and hypokalemic metabolic alkalosis. Most of these consequences are discussed in Chaps. 5–7. Renal salt wasting is quite obvious given the fact that the thick ascending limb is responsible for the reabsorption of such a large percentage of the filtered load of NaCl. Additionally however, as we shall see later in this chapter, the volume depletion that occurs in this condition probably results from the inability of the kidney to reabsorb water efficiently from the collecting tubule.

Bartter's syndrome is caused by a defect in the $Na^+-K^+-2Cl^-$-cotransporter in the luminal membrane of the thick ascending limb.

REABSORPTION IN THE EARLY DISTAL TUBULE

Functionally, the distal tubule can be divided into an "early" and "late" segment. The early distal tubule exhibits fundamental transport characteristics that are similar to those of the ascending limb, namely that it is essentially impermeable to water but is capable of reabsorbing NaCl (Fig. 4-13). As in other nephron segments, the driving force for NaCl reabsorption is the basolateral Na^+-K^+-ATPase. In this segment, however, transport across the luminal membrane is mediated by an electroneutral Na^+-Cl^--symporter, which can be inhibited by a separate class of diuretic drugs known as the thiazides (e.g., hydrochlorothiazide).

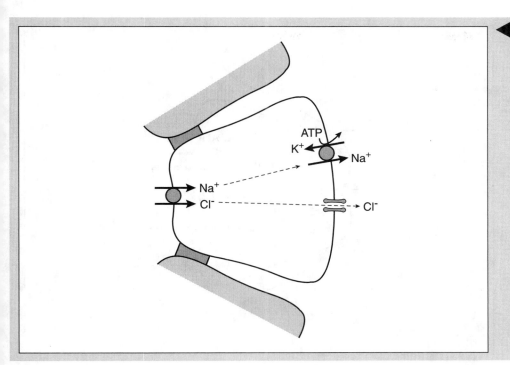

FIGURE 4-13
NaCl Reabsorption by the Early Distal Tubule. The luminal membrane Na^+–Cl^--cotransporter is inhibited by thiazide diuretics.

REABSORPTION IN THE LATE DISTAL TUBULE AND COLLECTING TUBULE

The cellular morphology as well as the permeability characteristics of the late distal tubule are similar to those of the collecting tubule system and thus are described together. Indeed they are often referred to collectively as the "distal nephron." These nephron segments possess two distinct cell types known as the principal cell and the intercalated cell. The principal cells are responsible for the reabsorption of NaCl and water and for the secretion of K^+. The intercalated cells are primarily involved in the secretion of H^+ (see Chap. 7) but also have a limited capacity for reabsorption of K^+. The transport of Na^+ across the luminal membrane of principal cells is facilitated by Na^+-selective channels (see Chap. 2, Fig. 2-9). The concomitant reabsorption of Cl^- that occurs in this segment is probably primarily paracellular and is driven by the lumen-negative potential that results from the primary transcellular transport of Na^+. Reabsorption can be inhibited in this segment by a group of diuretics including amiloride and triamterene, which act by blocking the luminal Na^+ channel.

An important factor in this distal nephron is that the reabsorption of both Na^+ and water is under hormonal control. Specifically, the mineralocorticoid aldosterone stimulates reabsorption of Na^+ particularly in the cortical collecting tubule, while the neurohypophyseal peptide antidiuretic hormone (ADH) stimulates water reabsorption along the entire length of this distal nephron. The fundamental intracellular mechanisms used by these two hormones have now been established, although some details have yet to be clarified.

> The late distal and collecting tubule contain principal and intercalated cells.

Aldosterone and Sodium Chloride Reabsorption

Aldosterone is secreted from the zona glomerulosa cells of the adrenal cortex and acts in a classic steroid hormone fashion, by stimulating protein synthesis. In this instance, aldosterone binds to intracellular receptors and is thought to stimulate the synthesis of several proteins that play a key role in the Na^+ reabsorptive process including the basolateral membrane Na^+–K^+-ATPase and the luminal membrane Na^+-selective channel (Fig. 4-14). In addition, it is likely that aldosterone also stimulates the production of

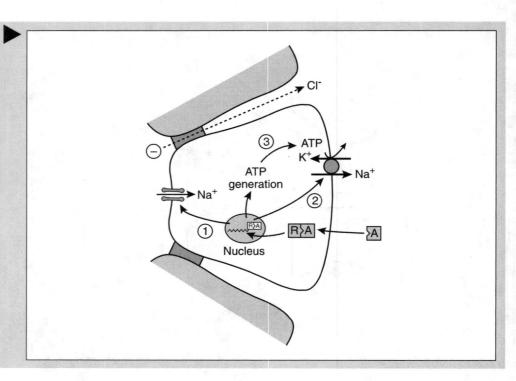

FIGURE 4-14 ▶

Intracellular Mechanism of Action of Aldosterone (A) in the Collecting Tubule. The lipophilic hormone freely traverses the plasma membrane and binds to cytoplasmic receptors (R), which then enter the nucleus and trigger transcription of several genes, including those for the luminal membrane Na⁺ channel (1); the basolateral membrane Na⁺–K⁺-ATPase (2); and Krebs cycle enzymes involved in adenosine triphosphate (ATP) synthesis (3).

Aldosterone stimulates NaCl reabsorption in the cortical collecting tubule.

several Krebs cycle enzymes, thereby facilitating the increased production of adenosine triphosphate (ATP) for the Na⁺–K⁺ pump. Quantitatively, aldosterone can determine the fate of 5%–6% of the filtered load of Na⁺, which translates to approximately 1250 mEq/d. In the complete absence of aldosterone then, the Na⁺ escapes reabsorption and, thus, is for the most part excreted. At first glance, the loss of such a relatively small percentage of the filtered load of Na⁺ might be considered to have relatively little potential impact on overall body fluid homeostasis. This is in fact not the case. When one considers that each liter of extracellular fluid (ECF) contains approximately 140 mEq of Na⁺, the principles discussed in Chap. 1 should make it apparent that the loss of 1250 mEq of Na⁺ will have profound effects on body fluid volume and osmolarity. This issue will be discussed in more detail in Chap. 5.

Antidiuretic Hormone and Water Reabsorption

ADH is a peptide hormone that is released from the posterior pituitary. ADH uses the intracellular second messenger cyclic adenosine monophosphate (cAMP) to increase water permeability of the distal nephron (Fig. 4-15). In this pathway, ADH binds to receptors located on the basolateral membrane, resulting in the activation of the enzyme adenylate cyclase and the subsequent generation of cAMP from ATP. Transepithelial transport of water in a number of nephron segments is facilitated by specific water channels known as aquaporins. In "upstream" nephron segments such as the proximal tubule and thin descending limb of the loop of Henle, aquaporins are constitutively expressed and permanently embedded within the luminal and basolateral membranes of the cell. In the case of the collecting tubule, however, *luminal* membrane water channels can be selectively inserted and retrieved, thereby altering the overall water permeability of this segment. This process basically uses the principals of exocytosis and endocytosis. Water channels either exist embedded in the luminal membrane or associated with vesicles within the cytoplasm. Under conditions of low-circulating ADH levels, most vesicles are associated with these vesicles. Increased production of ADH stimulates cAMP production, which, via a cascade of events that has yet to be fully defined, results in the fusion of vesicles with the luminal membrane in a manner similar to that which occurs during exocytosis (see Fig. 4-15). As a result, water channels are effectively "inserted" into this membrane, resulting in increased water permeability. As plasma ADH levels decrease, cAMP production declines and results in the recovery of water

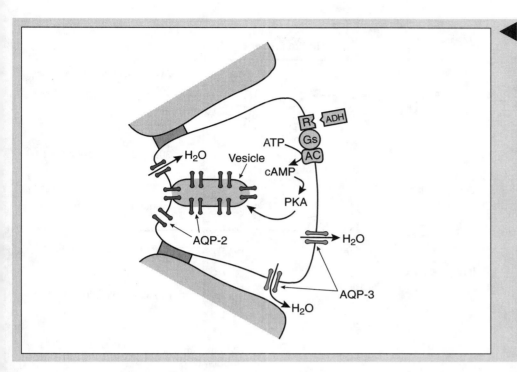

FIGURE 4-15
Intracellular Mechanism of Action of Anti-diuretic Hormone (ADH) in the Collecting Tubule. ADH binds to a basolateral membrane stimulatory G protein (Gs)–coupled receptor (R), resulting in the activation of adenylate cyclase (AC) and synthesis of cyclic adenosine monophosphate (cAMP). The subsequent activation of protein kinase A (PKA) ultimately leads to the incorporation of cytosolic vesicle-associated water channels (AQP-2) into the luminal membrane. Note that a distinct water channel isoform (AQP-3) is constitutively associated with the basolateral membrane.

channels from the luminal membrane by a process similar to endocytosis. In this case, however, endocytosed channels are not ultimately degraded but rather are held within the cytosol until membrane reinsertion can occur when ADH levels rise again. It is important to note that this process only affects water channel insertion into the luminal membrane. Water channels are permanently associated with the basolateral membrane. You will recall that aquaporin-1 (AQP-1) is expressed in the proximal and thin descending limb segments. Intriguingly, it appears that it is aquaporin-2 (AQP-2) that is "shuttled" in and out of the luminal membrane of the collecting tubule, while aquaporin-3 and probably aquaporin-4 (AQP-3, AQP-4) are constitutively expressed in the basolateral membrane of these cells.

The water permeability of the luminal membrane of the collecting tubule can be varied by the selective insertion and retrieval of water channels. This process is regulated by ADH.

As in the thin descending limb, the reabsorption of water is dependent on the existence of an osmotic gradient from lumen to interstitium. Under most conditions, this gradient exists along the entire length of the distal nephron. Recall that as a result of selective reabsorption of NaCl in the ascending limb of the loop of Henle, fluid entering the distal nephron is hypotonic ($\approx$ 100 mOsm/L). Consequently, as the fluid flows through the late distal and cortical collecting tubule a 100 $\rightarrow$ 300 mOsm/L (in $\rightarrow$ out) osmotic gradient initially exists, which in the presence of ADH will drive water reabsorption. Tubular fluid that flows from the cortex into the medullary collecting tubule can, therefore, achieve a maximal osmolarity of 300 mOsm/L; that is, it achieves osmotic equilibrium with the cortical interstitium (Fig. 4-16). As the tubular fluid flows down the medullary collecting tubule toward the papilla, it continues to be concentrated as more water is reabsorbed as a result of the progressive increase in medullary interstitial osmolarity. At the tip of the papillary collecting duct, therefore, the osmolarity of the tubular fluid in humans can increase to 1200–1400 mOsm/L corresponding to the maximal osmolarity of the interstitium. A rat, on the other hand, can concentrate urine to 3000–3500 mOsm/L because interstitial osmolarity at the tip of the papilla in this species is 3000–3500 mOsm/L.

One misconception often arises when considering water reabsorption by the collecting tubule. Many individuals will perhaps predict that with high plasma ADH levels, a greater volume of water is reabsorbed from the medullary and papillary collecting tubules than from the cortical collecting tubules. Typically, the reasoning is based on the fact that this must be so since the osmolarity of the tubular fluid increases to a much greater extent along the medullary (300 $\rightarrow$ 1200 mOsm/L) as compared to the cortical collecting tubule (100 $\rightarrow$ 300 mOsm/L). In fact, this is not correct. Consider the volume of fluid delivered to each segment. Approximately 10% (18 L) of the filtered load of water is

FIGURE 4-16 ▶
Effect of Antidiuretic Hormone (ADH) on Urine Osmolarity as a Result of Water Reabsorption by the Collecting Tubule System.

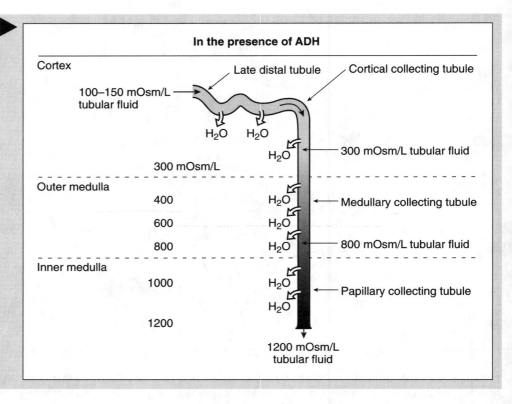

In the presence of ADH

The renal response to an increase in ADH will occur more quickly than the response to an increase in aldosterone, since the latter mechanism requires de novo protein synthesis.

delivered to the distal nephron. To elevate the osmolarity of this tubular fluid from approximately $100 \rightarrow 300$ mOsm/L, the volume must be reduced by two-thirds; that is, 12 L of water must be reabsorbed by the cortical collecting tubule. Subsequently, to raise the osmolarity of this tubular fluid from $300 \rightarrow 1200$ mOsm/L, the volume must be reduced by three-fourths. Since only 6 L are delivered to the medullary collecting tubule, this translates to the reabsorption of only 4.5 L of water. Contrary to what might be predicted then, in the presence of ADH, a greater volume of water is in fact reabsorbed from the cortical collecting tubule than from more distal collecting tubular segments.

Consider the other extreme. In the absence of ADH and thus the absence of luminal membrane water channels, the entire cortical and medullary collecting tubule system is essentially impermeable to water despite the continued presence of a favorable osmotic gradient in $\rightarrow$ out. However, the distal nephron is still capable of reabsorbing Na^+, which creates an even more dilute tubular fluid. Consequently, in a human, the absence of ADH results in the excretion of a large volume of very dilute, hypotonic (50–75 mOsm/L) urine.

One last issue deserves consideration in this section. Aldosterone and ADH often work together to maintain a constant body fluid volume and osmolarity. It should be apparent from their respective modes of action described earlier, that they must operate on quite different time frames. Fundamentally, <u>ADH acts much more quickly than aldosterone</u>. For ADH, the generation of cAMP, the subsequent insertion of water channels into the luminal membrane, and thus the increase in water reabsorption are quite rapid, probably in the order of a few minutes. In contrast, the predominant mechanism of action of aldosterone requires *de novo* protein synthesis. Consequently, a significant increase in Na^+ reabsorption in response to aldosterone is likely to take many minutes to hours.

COUNTERCURRENT MULTIPLICATION SYSTEM

Deposition of NaCl

Having reviewed the transport characteristics of nephron segments beyond the proximal tubule, it is now possible to appreciate the mechanism by which the hypertonic medullary interstitium is generated. The center of the process is countercurrent multiplication, which basically is a very energy-efficient means by which NaCl can be selectively deposited within the renal medulla. The thick ascending limb of the loop of Henle reabsorbs NaCl without concomitant water reabsorption. As in all transport processes, there is a maximal transepithelial concentration gradient that can be maintained by this transport process. In the thick ascending limb, the prevailing transport mechanism for NaCl is able to maintain a 200 mOsm/L concentration difference between the tubular fluid (lower) and the interstitium. At this point, the system is in a steady state where the rate of flux of NaCl from lumen to interstitium is matched by the rate of passive diffusion or back flux of NaCl from interstitium to lumen. Given this limitation, it would be impossible to generate a markedly hypertonic medullary interstitium containing high NaCl concentrations if only isotonic (300 mOsm/L) fluid were delivered to the ascending limb. This in fact does not occur; rather, as a result of the selective water permeability of the thin descending limb, the overall concentration (and most importantly, NaCl concentration) of tubular fluid entering the ascending limb is high.

The traditional conceptual model used to illustrate countercurrent multiplication is presented in Fig. 4-17. The starting point is to assume that the entire loop of Henle

> The process of countercurrent multiplication is responsible for the selective deposition of NaCl within the renal medulla.

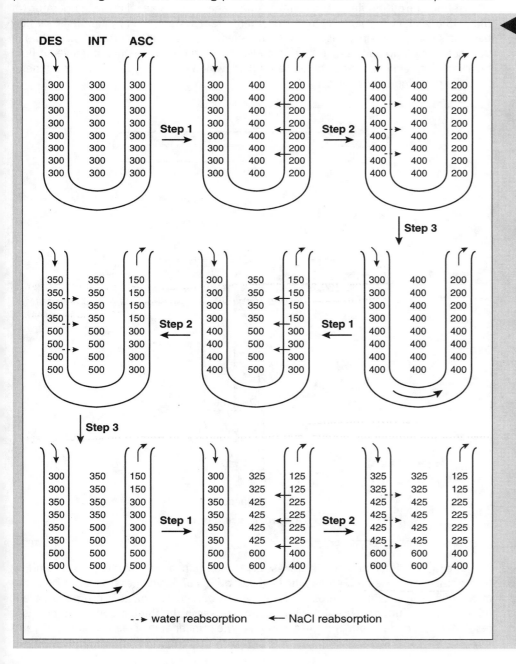

◄ FIGURE 4-17
Loop of Henle and Countercurrent Multiplication. *This is a conceptual presentation of the mechanism by which NaCl is deposited in the medullary interstitium (INT). Beginning with a loop containing isotonic fluid and an isotonic medulla, the repetition of three sequential steps ultimately generates a vertical medullary interstitial osmotic gradient. Step 1 is reabsorption of NaCl by the ascending limb (ASC); step 2 is reabsorption of water from the thin descending limb (DES); and step 3 is fluid flow and delivery of more isotonic fluid into the loop from the proximal tubule.*

contains isotonic fluid and that the medullary interstitium is also isotonic. Three sequential processes must then occur repeatedly to generate a linear hypertonic gradient within the medulla. In step 1, NaCl is reabsorbed from the thick ascending limb until a 200 mOsm/L gradient has been established between the tubular fluid and the interstitium. In step 2, the hypertonic interstitium stimulates the reabsorption of water from the thin descending limb, which creates an equally hypertonic tubular fluid in this segment. In step 3, flow occurs within the loop so that more isotonic fluid enters the loop from the proximal tubule, and hypertonic fluid generated in the thin descending limb is delivered to the ascending limb. Steps 1–3 are then repeated multiple times. The end result is that a large vertical osmotic gradient has been generated within the medullary interstitium, yet no more than a 200 mOsm/L gradient exists between the interstitium and ascending limb fluid at any horizontal level. It should be apparent that the deposition of NaCl within the medullary interstitium is dependent on the unique permeability characteristics of both the ascending and descending limbs of the loop of Henle. This countercurrent multiplication system is often compared to a heat exchanger, where flow in opposite directions of two closely juxtaposed tubes results in preheating of input fluid by transfer of heat from the output fluid. As a result, a single heat source can raise the temperature of the fluid to a much higher level in this countercurrent system, than by simple linear flow past the same heat source (Fig. 4-18). In the medulla, the countercurrent flow of fluid in the ascending limb and descending limb results not in the preheating of delivered fluid but rather in *preconcentration* of delivered fluid, which ultimately facilitates the generation of a hypertonic renal medulla.

FIGURE 4-18 ▶

Heat Exchanger Analogy. In a countercurrent heat exchanger, the input fluid is preheated by transferring heat from the output fluid. This arrangement results in a much greater increase in fluid temperature than could be accomplished by simple linear flow of fluid past the same heat source. By analogy, in the loop of Henle, fluid into the descending limb is preconcentrated, allowing more solute to be transported into the medullary interstitium than could be accomplished if isotonic fluid were delivered to this segment.

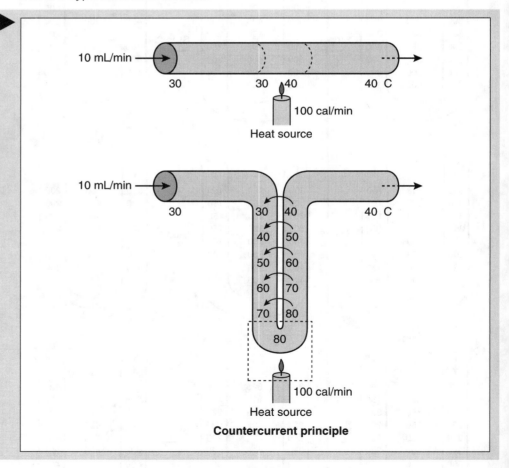

The rate-limiting step in countercurrent multiplication is reabsorption of NaCl by the thick ascending limb of the loop of Henle.

The rate-limiting step in this process is reabsorption of NaCl by the thick ascending limb of the loop of Henle. Perhaps the best illustration of this comes from examining the effect of the loop diuretic furosemide. As we discussed earlier, this drug is a potent inhibitor of the luminal $Na^+–K^+–2Cl^-$-cotransporter in the thick ascending limb. As a result of furosemide treatment, the ascending limb is incapable of reabsorbing NaCl, and over time the medullary interstitial osmolarity decreases. As this occurs, less water can be reabsorbed from the descending limb, and thus concentration of tubular fluid decreases. In the extreme, therefore, the medullary interstitium will become isotonic, and tubular fluid exiting the loop of Henle will be isotonic, that is essentially the same as was delivered to the loop out of the proximal tubule. You may recall that this condition is identical to the starting conditions used to illustrate the process of countercurrent multiplication. Physiologically, restoration of the hypertonic interstitium involves all three steps described earlier, but in reality they occur simultaneously rather than sequentially as proposed in the model. Pathophysiologically, any condition that depresses NaCl reabsorption by the thick ascending limb will also affect concentrating ability. Two such examples were presented earlier in this chapter. Adrenal insufficiency impairs loop transport and is associated with an inability to dilute or concentrate the urine. Similarly, Bartter's syndrome is characterized by volume depletion as a result of excessive urine output.

Deposition of Urea

In addition to the deposition of NaCl, the hypertonicity of the renal medulla is also dependent on the selective deposition of urea. The mechanism underlying the deposition of urea is totally different from that for NaCl. However, it does depend on specific transport characteristics of distal nephron segments, in particular differential urea permeability along the length of the collecting tubule. Although the two mechanisms are very different, they are dependent on one another for optimal activity. Urea really is a metabolic waste product, and there is no question that one responsibility of the kidney is to excrete urea. However, a percentage of the filtered load of urea is put to good use within the medulla. One illustration of the importance of urea to the renal concentrating mechanism is that subjects placed on a low-protein diet exhibit a reduced concentrating ability. The major reason for this deficit is that a reduced protein intake results in reduced protein catabolism and thus reduced urea generation and renal medullary deposition.

The key components of this process occur in the collecting tubule. As presented in Fig. 4-19, approximately 50% of the filtered load of urea is reabsorbed in the proximal tubule. The remainder is delivered to the distal tubule. Most importantly, the cortical and outer medullary collecting tubules are essentially impermeable to urea. Thus, in the presence of ADH, water reabsorption progressively increases the tubular fluid concentra-

> *Urea is reabsorbed predominantly by the inner medullary collecting tubule.*

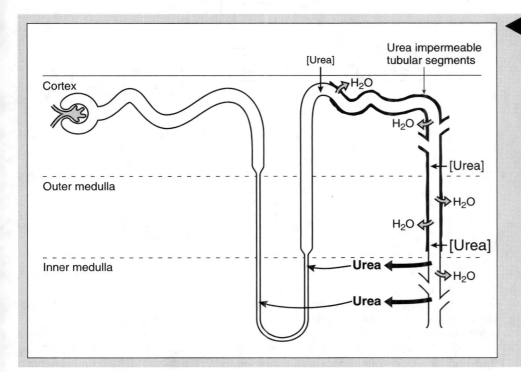

◀ **FIGURE 4-19**
Mechanism of Urea Deposition in the Inner Medulla. *The cortical and outer medullary collecting tubules are impermeable to urea. In the presence of antidiuretic hormone (ADH), the tubular fluid urea concentration increases sufficiently to promote passive reabsorption out of the inner medullary collecting tubule. Some urea deposited in the medullary interstitium passively diffuses into the lumen of the thin descending and ascending limb of the loop of Henle.*

tion of urea. In contrast to the cortical and outer medullary collecting tubules, basal urea permeability of the inner medullary collecting tubule is high due to the presence of specific urea transport proteins. Indeed, this transport process can be further enhanced in the presence of ADH. Consequently, at this point in the nephron, the tubular fluid urea concentration is sufficiently high to create a favorable chemical gradient for reabsorption of urea into the surrounding medullary interstitium.

Given this high prevailing interstitial urea concentration, it is perhaps not surprising that some can diffuse into the lumen of both the thin descending and ascending limb of the loop of Henle (Fig. 4-19). In the presence of ADH, however, this does not result in a net loss of medullary urea, since it will simply be reconcentrated within the early collecting tubule system and be reabsorbed out of the inner medullary collecting tubule. However, if ADH levels are low, water permeability of the collecting tubule will be low (see Fig. 4-20). Thus, the tubular fluid urea concentration does not rise to the level required for passive reabsorption, and as a result, more urea is excreted in the urine. Over time the medullary interstitial urea concentration and therefore osmolarity decreases. This is not detrimental to overall renal function however, when one takes into account that ADH levels should be low because total body water is inappropriately high. As we shall see in Chapter 5, the renal response to re-establish homeostasis is to increase water excretion, and this occurs by decreasing water reabsorption in the collecting tubule. Hence, a maximally hypertonic interstitial medulla would not be required under these circumstances.

FIGURE 4-20 ▶

Effects of Antidiuretic Hormone (ADH) on Medullary Interstitial Deposition of Urea and NaCl and as a Result, Medullary Osmolarity.

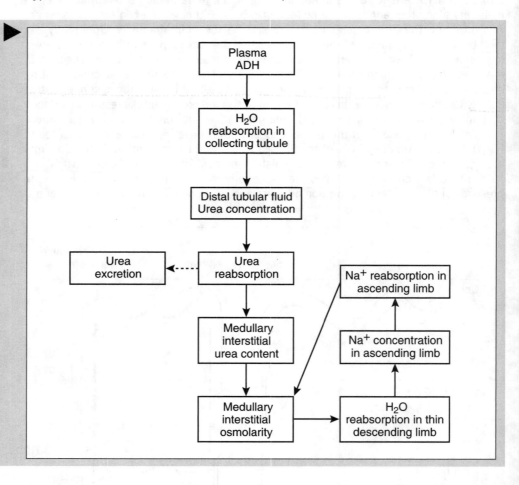

Under the conditions of reduced ADH levels, the deposition of NaCl as well as urea will decrease and therefore contribute to the reduced total medullary interstitial osmolarity. This will occur because when urea reabsorption declines, the concomitant decrease in medullary osmolarity will decrease the extent to which water can be reabsorbed by the thin descending limb, and thus the extent to which tubular fluid in the descending limb can be concentrated. As a result, presentation of tubular fluid with a lower NaCl concentration to the ascending limb reduces the capacity for NaCl reabsorption and thus deposition within the medulla.

Maintenance of Hypertonic Medullary Interstitium: Countercurrent Exchange

In Chap. 2, we emphasized that the renal medulla contained a unique network of capillaries referred to as the vasa recta. These capillaries originate from the efferent arterioles of juxtamedullary nephrons and typically exhibit a hairpin loop configuration, descending to varying depths into the medulla and thus running in parallel with the loops of Henle. This unique arrangement, coupled with a slow rate of blood flow through the capillaries, is essential for the maintenance of the hypertonic medullary interstitium. As with all other tissues, the renal medulla must be perfused with blood in order to supply oxygen and vital nutrients, as well as to remove metabolic waste products. Additionally, however, there must be a peritubular capillary system within the medulla to receive reabsorbed water and solute. The vasa recta subserve all of these functions but do so without destroying the hypertonic interstitium, which could occur if the medulla were supplied with a diffuse capillary network such as occurs within the renal cortex.

Consider the following problem (Fig. 4-21). Plasma entering the medulla from the cortex is, by definition, an isotonic fluid. As this fluid descends into the medulla, the marked differences in osmolarity and composition of the capillary fluid and interstitium result in diffusion of solute into and osmotic flux of water out of the capillaries. If this situation was not reversed in some way, the hypertonic medullary gradient would be rapidly destroyed. The vasa recta in fact prevent this from happening. In the descending vasa recta, the shifts in solute and water described above do indeed occur, such that at the tip of a capillary loop, the plasma can be extremely hypertonic (see Fig. 4-21). Now, however, plasma flows back toward the cortex, and thus flows through an environment of progressively decreasing tonicity. Consequently, the flux of solute and water is effectively reversed, and the medullary interstitial gradient is thereby maintained. This process is often referred to as countercurrent exchange.

> Countercurrent exchange occurs in the vasa recta and helps preserve the hypertonic medullary interstitium.

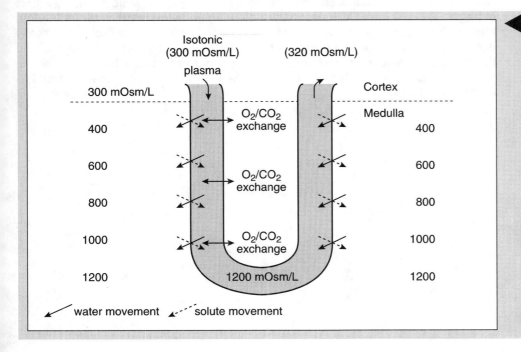

water movement   solute movement

◄ FIGURE 4-21
Vasa Recta and Countercurrent Exchange. *Isotonic plasma delivered from the cortex becomes progressively more hypertonic as it flows down the descending vasa recta into the deeper sections of the medulla. This occurs as a result of osmotic efflux of water into the hypertonic interstitium, and diffusion of interstitial solute into the capillary. As plasma flows back toward the cortex, this flux of solute and water is reversed, since the hypertonicity of the medullary interstitium progressively decreases. This countercurrent flow allows the normal transcapillary exchange of essential nutrients, metabolic waste products and O_2–CO_2 while preserving the hypertonic interstitium.*

As these fluxes are occurring, oxygen and nutrients are delivered to, and carbon dioxide and waste products removed from, the medullary tissue. A low plasma flow rate is essential to this process, to allow sufficient time for equilibration to occur across the capillary, particularly during the ascending phase. An inappropriate rise in the rate of medullary blood flow can lead to a breakdown in the interstitial osmotic gradient, a condition referred to as medullary washout. Under normal circumstances, it is important to understand that the volume and composition of plasma entering and exiting the medulla are not identical. In fact, the exiting volume (flow rate) and solute content (osmolarity) are significantly higher. This difference reflects the amount of water reabsorbed by the thin descending limbs and medullary collecting tubules, and the amount of solute (particularly NaCl) that is reabsorbed by the medullary thick ascending limb over and above that which is required to maintain the hypertonic environment.

RESOLUTION OF CLINICAL CASE

The patient suffered a myocardial infarction with two consequences. First, the diminished ability of the heart to pump blood led to accumulation of fluid in the lungs and resulted in pulmonary edema. Because of decreased cardiac output and underperfusion of the body, the activity of the sympathetic nervous system was increased, leading to a vasoconstriction of the systemic circulation, including the kidneys. Along with other physiologic mechanisms, the renal constriction and decreased GFR resulted in retention of both Na^+ and water. Thus, in the first few hours following the heart attack, the patient excreted a relatively small volume of concentrated urine containing very little Na^+. Treatment with furosemide decreased the ability of the thick ascending limb of the loop of Henle to reabsorb Na^+ and resulted in a marked increase in Na^+ excretion in spite of the low-sodium intake. An additional consequence of the decreased ability of the thick ascending limb to transport Na^+ is a decreased ability to concentrate the urine. A hypertonic renal medulla is necessary for water reabsorption from the medullary collecting duct, and the medullary hypertonicity is critically dependent on the deposition of NaCl into the medulla from the thick ascending limb. If NaCl is not deposited into the medulla, the medullary osmolarity dissipates, and the osmotic gradient both for water and subsequent urea reabsorption from the medullary collecting duct is lost. In this condition, the kidney cannot concentrate the urine to any appreciable extent regardless of the circulating levels of ADH. Hence, the loop diuretic decreased thick ascending limb transport and resulted in increased Na^+ excretion in a relatively large volume of nearly isotonic urine. After discontinuing the diuretic treatment, loop transport returned, and the medullary gradient was restored. The kidneys were again able to concentrate the urine and maintain normal Na^+ balance as indicated by the data obtained in the final 24-hour urine collection.

REVIEW QUESTIONS

1. Which one of the following statements is correct?

    (A) The effect of antidiuretic hormone (ADH) has a slower onset time than the effect of aldosterone.

    (B) The stimulatory effect of aldosterone on Na^+ reabsorption is due in part to increased Na^+-K^+-ATPase activity.

    (C) Reabsorption of all of the filtered Na^+ requires luminal membrane cotransporter proteins.

    (D) Aldosterone can regulate the reabsorption of up to 20% of the filtered load of Na^+.

2. Which of the following statements concerning the proximal tubule is true?

    (A) The filtered load of glucose normally exceeds the T_m for glucose.

    (B) Net reabsorption is increased when peritubular capillary hydrostatic and oncotic pressures are increased.

    (C) The *osmolarity* of the tubular fluid at the beginning and end of the proximal tubule is identical, but the *composition* of the fluid may be very different at these two sites.

    (D) Cl^- is the primary anion reabsorbed with Na^+ in the early proximal tubule.

3. Which one of the following combinations would best describe the tubular fluid concentration at various points along a human long-looped nephron in the absence of antidiuretic hormone (ADH)?

	End Proximal	End Thin Descending Limb	End Thick Ascending Limb	Final Urine
(A)	300 mOsm/L	1200 mOsm/L	300 mOsm/L	100 mOsm/L
(B)	300	600	100	1200
(C)	300	600	120	50
(D)	300	600	50	1200

4. Which one of the following statements is correct?

    (A) Loop diuretics inhibit the Na^+-K^+-ATPase on the basolateral membrane of the thick ascending limb cell.

    (B) In the thick ascending limb, paracellular (between cell) reabsorption of several cations is dependent on reflux of K^+ via luminal membrane K^+ channels.

    (C) The thin descending limb is often referred to as the "diluting segment."

    (D) The volume of water reabsorbed by the thin descending limb is identical during diuresis and antidiuresis.

5. Which one of the following statements is correct?

    (A) Aquaporin-2 (AQP-2) is located in the luminal membrane of proximal tubule, thin descending limb, and collecting tubule cells.

    (B) The effect of antidiuretic hormone (ADH) on water permeability of the collecting tubule is dependent on de novo protein synthesis.

    (C) Reabsorption of NaCl by the thick ascending limb is the rate-limiting step in countercurrent multiplication.

    (D) In maximal antidiuresis, urine flow ceases completely.

6. Urea recycling has which of the following characteristics?
   (A) It requires a urea-impermeable inner medullary collecting tubule.
   (B) It increases in the absence of antidiuretic hormone (ADH).
   (C) It participates in the generation of an hypertonic medullary interstitium.
   (D) It involves reabsorption of urea from the thin descending and thin ascending limb of the loop of Henle.

ANSWERS AND EXPLANATIONS

1. **The answer is B.** The aldosterone-dependent increase in Na^+-K^+-ATPase activity will tend to lower intracellular Na^+ concentration. As a result the chemical concentration gradient for Na^+ entry into the cell across the luminal membrane is increased. This increased ion flux is probably also facilitated by an aldosterone-dependent increase in the synthesis of luminal membrane Na^+ selective channels. Option A is incorrect. A peptide hormone such as ADH utilizes the intracellular second messenger cAMP to trigger the insertion of water channels into the luminal membrane of collecting tubule cells. This response can occur within seconds to minutes. In contrast, the action of the steroid hormone aldosterone is dependent on the synthesis of new proteins that can take several hours. Option C is incorrect. It is true that the reabsorption of much of the Na^+ in the proximal tubule is mediated via Na^+-coupled co-transporters, such as Na^+-glucose, phosphate, amino-acid, etc. Additionally, reabsorption of much of the Na^+ in the thick ascending limb of the loop of Henle is mediated by a unique luminal membrane Na^+-K^+ 2 Cl co-transporter. However, as presented above in the collecting tubule, a considerable percentage of luminal membrane transport occurs via Na^+-selective channels. Additionally, some Na^+ reabsorption occurs paracellularly, particularly in the proximal tubule and thick ascending limb. Option D is incorrect. It is absolutely correct that aldosterone can regulate the reabsorption of Na^+. It is not correct, however, that aldosterone has control over the reabsorption of 20% of the filtered load of Na^+. The principal site of action of aldosterone is the cortical collecting tubule, and by the time the filtrate reaches this point, approximately 90% of the filtered load of Na^+ has already been reabsorbed. In actuality, aldosterone regulates the reabsorption of perhaps 5–8% of this remaining 10% of the filtered load.

2. **The answer is C.** Tubular fluid at both the beginning and end of the proximal tubule is essentially isotonic ($\approx$ 290 mOsm/L). However, as a result of water reabsorption, at the end of the proximal tubule, the total volume of tubular fluid has been reduced by two-thirds, and as a result of a combination of reabsorption and secretion, the solute composition of this fluid has been altered dramatically. As one example, all of the filtered glucose is reabsorbed along the proximal tubule, since the amount filtered is much less that the maximal reabsorptive capacity. Hence option A is incorrect. Option B is also incorrect because an increase in peritubular colloid osmotic pressure would indeed favor increased reabsorption; however, an increase in peritubular capillary hydrostatic pressure would oppose rather than promote reabsorption. Option D is incorrect because Cl^- is predominantly reabsorbed with Na^+ in the late rather than the early proximal tubule.

3. **The answer is C.** To answer this question, it is important to appreciate the following. First, in the absence of ADH, water cannot be reabsorbed from the collecting tubule; therefore, urine cannot be concentrated. Hence, options B and D must be incorrect. Second, if water reabsorption from the collecting tubule is minimal, urea cannot be reabsorbed from the papillary collecting tubule; therefore, the renal medullary interstitial osmolarity decreases. As a result, fluid in the descending limb of the loop of

Henle cannot be concentrated to the maximal extent of 1200–1400 mOsm/L in the human kidney. Therefore, option A must be incorrect. The one value that is relatively independent of the state of water balance is the osmolality of tubular fluid in the proximal tubule. Under all conditions, isotonic fluid is generated within this nephron segment.

4. **The answer is B.** Several cations including Na^+, K^+, Ca^{2+}, and Mg^{2+} are reabsorbed paracellularly in the thick ascending limb. The primary driving force for this movement across the tight junctions is the lumen-positive potential. This potential in turn is generated as a result of reflux of K^+ across the luminal membrane via K^+-selective channels. This K^+ entered the cell via the Na^+–K^+–$2Cl^-$-cotransporter. Option A is incorrect because loop diuretics such as furosemide or bumetanide inhibit the Na^+–K^+–$2Cl^-$-cotransporter on the luminal membrane of the thick ascending limb cell. Option C is incorrect because it is the *ascending* limb of the loop of Henle that is referred to as the diluting segment. Since the thick ascending limb is able to reabsorb NaCl but is totally impermeable to water, the hypertonic tubular fluid that enters this segment from the thin descending limb is progressively diluted to the extent that as it enters the early distal convoluted tubule, it is typically very hypotonic (≈ 100 mOsm/L). Option D is incorrect because the extent to which tubular fluid is concentrated in the thin descending limb is dependent on the prevailing osmotic gradient within the renal medulla. In the absence of ADH (diuresis), the ability to reabsorb urea is reduced. As a result, urea deposition within the medulla and, thus osmolarity, decreases. This reduces the driving force for water reabsorption out of the thin descending limb.

5. **The answer is C.** Reabsorption of NaCl from the medullary thick ascending limb of the loop of Henle is central to the process of countercurrent multiplication. If this process is inhibited, for example, by loop diuretics, the hypertonicity of the renal medullary interstitium is markedly reduced. It deserves emphasis, however, that countercurrent multiplication per se also requires several additional factors to be effective, including a hairpin-loop configuration of the loops of Henle and specific permeability characteristics of the descending limb, ascending limb, and collecting tubular system. Option A is incorrect because interestingly, AQP-2 is currently thought to be exclusively located in the luminal membrane of the collecting tubule system. This water channel, therefore, is also unique in being the only one that can be selectively inserted and retrieved from a cell membrane. This response is controlled by ADH. Mechanistically, the peptide hormone ADH triggers this response via the generation of cAMP. This process does not require *de novo* protein synthesis, and therefore, option C is incorrect. However, it should be noted that there is now some evidence to suggest that ADH may stimulate AQP-2 mRNA transcription, which would ultimately result in increased synthesis of aquaporin protein. Option D is incorrect because even in maximal antidiuresis, urine flow will not stop, since the kidney is obligated to excrete metabolic waste products in solution. This can be achieved by excreting a minimum of 500 mL or so of urine a day in humans.

6. **The answer is C.** Urea recycling facilitates the deposition of urea within the renal medullary interstitium, thereby increasing medullary osmolarity. Option A is incorrect because it is the cortical (and outer medullary) collecting tubule that must be impermeable to urea so that in the presence of ADH, water reabsorption progressively concentrates urea within the tubular fluid. Once this fluid reaches the inner medullary collecting tubule, it has reached a sufficiently high concentration to be passively reabsorbed into the medullary interstitium. Based on this scenario, it is apparent that urea reabsorption will *decrease* in the absence of ADH since it will not be concentrated to the same extent. Therefore, option B is incorrect. Option D is also incorrect because urea recycling involves the passive diffusion of urea from the medullary interstitium *into* the lumen of the thin descending and ascending limb.

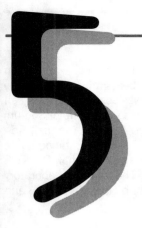

MAINTENANCE OF BODY FLUID OSMOLARITY AND VOLUME

CHAPTER OUTLINE

INTRODUCTION OF CLINICAL CASES

Case 1

A 60-year-old man presented at the emergency room complaining of periods of disorientation over the past several days. The patient history revealed that he was a heavy smoker and that he had gained almost 10 kg over the last 3–4 months. His physical examination revealed a blood pressure of 138/82 mm Hg and a pulse of 81 beats/min. A chest x-ray revealed a 5-cm mass in the upper right lobe. Sputum cytology was positive for small cell carcinoma. The following laboratory values were obtained from a serum sample: Sodium (Na^+), 110 mEq/L (normal, 136–145 mEq/L); chloride (Cl^-), 74 mEq/L (normal, 95–105 mEq/L); potassium (K^+), 4.0 mEq/L (normal, 3.5–5.1 mEq/L); bicarbonate (HCO_3^-), 22 mEq/L (normal, 21–29 mEq/L); creatinine, 1.1 mg/dL (normal, 0.5–1.5 mg/dL); and osmolarity, 225 mOsm/L (normal, 280 mOsm/L). The following laboratory values were obtained from a urine sample: volume, 500 mL/24 hr; Na^+, 78 mEq/L; and osmolarity, 504 mOsm/L.

Case 2

A 60-year-old man visited his physician complaining of ever increasing shortness of breath and pedal swelling. He found it increasingly difficult to ascend even one flight of stairs and was unable to lie flat in bed without becoming short of breath. The patient's history revealed angina and at least two documented myocardial infarctions. The patient had gained 10 kg over recent months. A physical examination revealed a blood pressure of 106/65 mm Hg and a pulse of 110 beats/min. There was a jugular venous distention of approximately 9 cm above the clavicle. The liver was enlarged, tender to the touch, and gentle pressure caused increased distension of the jugular veins. Laboratory data revealed a plasma creatinine concentration of 2 mg/dL and a urinary Na^+ concentration of 5 mEq/L.[1]

MAINTENANCE OF BODY FLUID OSMOLARITY

> Despite the profound differences in solute content of the intracellular and extracellular fluids, the osmolarity of these two fluids is identical (280–290 mOsm/L).

You will recall from Chap. 1 that the volumes as well as the solute content of the extracellular and intracellular fluids (ECF, ICF) are quite different. However, the osmolarity of these two fluids is identical and is typically maintained at 280–290 mOsm/L. The greatest threat to body fluid osmolarity is a net gain or loss of total body water. Typically, the insult initially affects ECF osmolarity. Given the water permeable nature of cell membranes, however, there must ultimately be an equal change in osmolarity of both ECF and ICF.

To illustrate this point, consider the effects of rapid ingestion of 1 L of pure water (Fig. 5-1). Prior to ingestion, ICF and ECF are isotonic. As this water load is absorbed from the gastrointestinal (GI) tract, it initially enters the ECF compartment. Since there is no concurrent change in solute absorption in this case, the osmolarity of the ECF must fall. Recalling principles discussed in Chap. 1, water now moves osmotically from this hypotonic ECF environment to the ICF compartment, until a new osmotic equilibrium is achieved. At this point, both the ECF and ICF volumes are *increased*, while the osmolarity of both are *decreased*, compared to the situation prior to ingestion of the water load. The homeostatic response to this water challenge is to reduce plasma antidiuretic hormone (ADH) levels, thus reducing water reabsorption by the collecting tubule and increasing water excretion. As the excess water is progressively removed from the ECF, osmolarity rises, thus causing efflux of water from the ICF to the ECF compartment. Ultimately, the 1 L of excess water is excreted, restoring the volume and osmolarity of both the ICF and ECF to normal. At the other extreme, a net loss of pure water from the body results in an increase in body fluid osmolarity. The homeostatic response to this situation involves two components. First, ADH levels increase, thereby increasing water reabsorption by the collecting tubule and minimizing water loss in the urine. Second, the thirst mechanism is stimulated, which provides a mechanism for rapidly replenishing the volume of water initially lost. It should be noted that the regulation of thirst is equally important in the excess water example. In that case, the thirst mechanism was suppressed to facilitate the net excretion of the 1 L of ingested water.

> Maintenance of total body water balance involves the regulation of both water excretion by the kidneys and regulation of water intake via the thirst mechanism.

---

1 Clinical cases adapted with permission from Shayman J: *Renal Pathophysiology*. Philadelphia, PA: J. B. Lippincott, 1995, pp 19, 49–50.

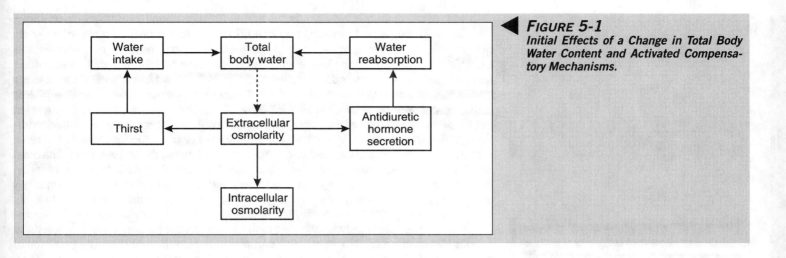

FIGURE 5-1
Initial Effects of a Change in Total Body Water Content and Activated Compensatory Mechanisms.

TOTAL BODY WATER BALANCE

The first part of this chapter focuses on the mechanisms involved in the regulation of ADH secretion and in the regulation of thirst. Before that, however, it is important to appreciate the factors that govern overall total body water balance and, therefore, body fluid osmolarity. As for many solutes and ions, total body water balance is maintained by matching water output to water intake. Fig. 5-2 illustrates the major routes of input and output. On the input side, water is ingested either as fluid or as a component of food, and a comparatively small volume of water can be generated metabolically. On the output side, there are several routes for water loss over which we have very little control, the so-called insensible water losses, which include the skin and lungs. Additionally, water can be lost in feces and by sweating. The actual volume lost can vary dramatically through these latter two routes. For example, fecal water losses increase during periods of diarrhea, while the volume of water lost in sweat increases as physical activity increases. However, neither system is homeostatically regulated and thus cannot contribute to the maintenance of water balance. In sharp contrast, urine output is tightly regulated and therefore is one of the primary contributors to maintaining water balance.

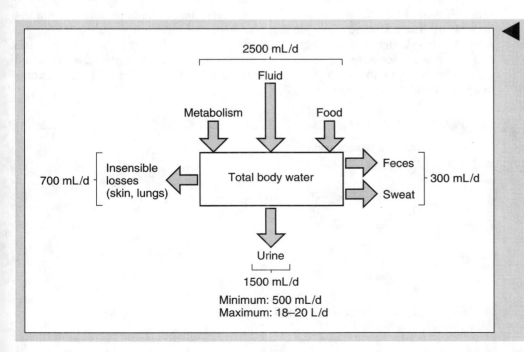

FIGURE 5-2
Routes of Water Input and Output in the Body. The values presented are for illustration only and vary from person to person and within any one individual depending on environmental conditions.

Consider the two extremes. Under conditions of water excess as a result of excess fluid intake, the renal response is to increase water excretion. In a state of maximal water excretion (maximal diuresis), urine volume can increase to 18–20 L/d. Two important facts should be emphasized. First, the volume of additional water excreted *exactly* matches the volume of excess water ingested. Second, the increased water excretion is *not* accompanied by increased solute excretion. Thus, the large volume of urine excreted in this particular example has a very low osmolarity. At the other extreme, under conditions of fluid depletion as a result of restricted intake or inappropriate losses, the renal response is to reduce water excretion. In a state of maximal conservation (maximal antidiuresis), urine volume can be reduced to as little as 500 mL/d. An initial reaction might be to ask why not reduce water output even further or perhaps shut it off completely and thereby conserve even more water. The reason that this cannot happen is that, as discussed in Chap. 1, the homeostatic responsibilities of the kidneys require the excretion of multiple solutes, including metabolic waste products, and various anions and cations. Since these solutes must be in solution, their excretion obligates the excretion of a minimum of 500 mL of water a day. Therefore, if urine output was reduced even further, the limited benefit of retaining additional water would be more than offset by the deleterious effects of impaired solute excretion on overall body fluid homeostasis.

> *Daily urine output can be as high as 20 L or as low as 500 mL.*

> *The need to excrete multiple solutes constantly obligates the kidneys to excrete a minimal volume of water, even under conditions that demand maximal water conservation.*

REGULATION OF ANTIDIURETIC HORMONE SECRETION

Synthesis and Secretion

> *ADH is synthesized in the cell bodies of magnocellular neurons located in the hypothalamus and released from axon terminals located in the posterior pituitary.*

The ability of the kidneys to excrete urine of variable volume and osmolarity is absolutely dependent on the action of ADH (Fig. 5-3). ADH is a nine amino acid peptide that is synthesized by magnocellular neurons of the supraoptic and paraventricular nuclei located in the hypothalamus. Once synthesized, ADH is packaged and transported to the axon terminals that are located in the posterior pituitary (neurohypophysis), where it is stored as insoluble complexes with carrier proteins known as neurophysins. Stimulation of these neurons leads to increased secretion of ADH into the capillary plexus of the efferent hypophysial vein and thus into the general circulation (Fig. 5-4). As in most other neurosecretory systems, the exocytotic release of ADH is dependent on a rise in intracellular calcium (Ca^{2+}), which results from the action potential–induced opening of voltage-gated Ca^{2+} channels. Prolonged stimulation eventually results in increased gene expression and therefore synthesis of ADH. However, this does not usually occur in the first 24–48 hours. Consequently, depletion of ADH stores can occur during this period when de novo synthesis fails to keep pace with secretion. In addition to ADH synthesis and secretion, a separate population of magnocellular neurons synthesizes a second peptide hormone, oxytocin, which is structurally quite similar to ADH but possesses only weak antidiuretic activity (see Fig. 5-3).

FIGURE 5-3 ▶

Structure of Arginine Vasopressin. The molecule consists of nine amino acids, but the disulfide bond between the cysteines at positions 1 and 6 effectively create an octapeptide. Substitution of leucine (Leu) for arginine at position 8 creates oxytocin, which is also synthesized and secreted by magnocellular neurons.

Arginine vasopressin

Cys — Tyr — Phe — Gln — Asn — Cys — Pro — Arg — Gly — NH₂
①   ⑨

Oxytocin

Cys — Tyr — Ile — Gln — Asn — Cys — Pro — Leu — Gly — NH₂
①   ⑨

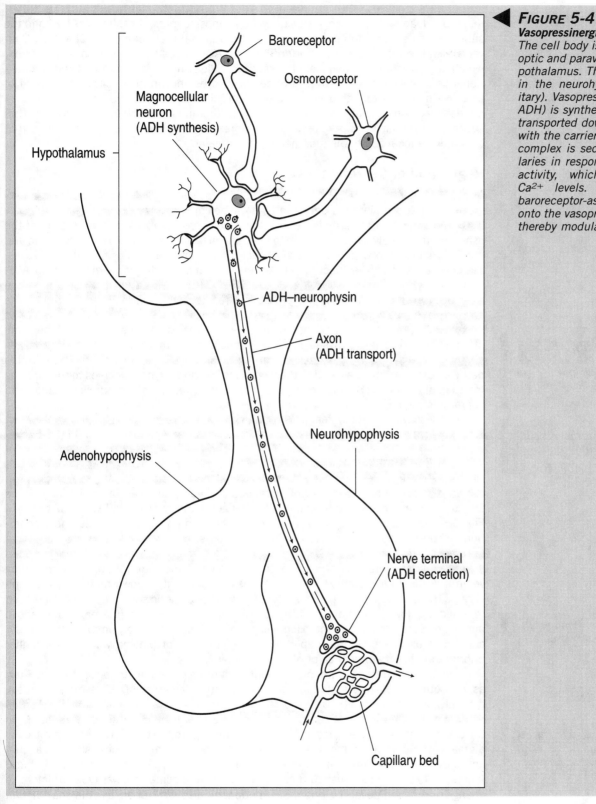

Baroreceptor

Osmoreceptor

Magnocellular
neuron
(ADH synthesis)

Hypothalamus

ADH–neurophysin

Axon
(ADH transport)

Neurohypophysis

Adenohypophysis

Nerve terminal
(ADH secretion)

Capillary bed

FIGURE 5-4
Vasopressinergic Magnocellular Neuron.
The cell body is located within the supra-optic and paraventricular nuclei of the hypothalamus. The axon terminal is located in the neurohypophysis (posterior pituitary). Vasopressin (antidiuretic hormone, ADH) is synthesized in the cell body and transported down the axon in association with the carrier protein neurophysin. This complex is secreted into adjacent capillaries in response to increased electrical activity, which increases intracellular Ca^{2+} levels. Both osmoreceptor- and baroreceptor-associated neurons synapse onto the vasopressinergic neuron and can thereby modulate ADH secretory activity.

It should be noted that many texts, including this one, alternately refer to ADH and arginine vasopressin (AVP). This latter designation is based on the fact that at higher, primarily supraphysiologic concentrations, ADH does in fact possess vasoconstrictor capacity. Mechanistically, this constrictor effect is mediated via an interaction with a distinct vasopressin receptor. In the collecting tubule, ADH binds to vasopressin V_2

receptors, leading to the generation of cyclic adenosine monophosphate (cAMP) and the subsequent translocation of aquaporins to the luminal membrane (see Chap. 4). Conversely, in the vascular system and in the liver, ADH binds to vasopressin V_1 receptors, which trigger phosphatidylinositol metabolism, leading to an inositol triphosphate–dependent release of Ca^{2+} from intracellular stores and, in many cases, activation of protein kinase C. Although beyond the scope of this text, it should be noted that the ever increasing complexity of signaling systems is further illustrated by current evidence that suggests that both V_1 and V_2 receptors are present on collecting tubule cells and that they may be localized to distinct membrane domains.

Regulation of Secretion

The rate of secretion of ADH is primarily dictated by the osmolarity of the ECF compartment. Plasma osmolarity is detected by a cluster of osmoreceptors located within the hypothalamus. As osmolarity increases, these cells presumably shrink as a result of the osmotic withdrawal of water, leading to the transmission of a signal to the supraoptic and paraventricular nuclei to increase ADH secretion. Conversely, as osmolarity decreases, the cells expand as they accumulate water, ultimately leading to a reduction in ADH secretion. ADH secretion can also be affected by changes in plasma volume. These changes are detected both by low-pressure baroreceptors located primarily in the atria and pulmonary veins and by high-pressure baroreceptors located in the carotid sinus and aortic arch. (An additional series of high-pressure baroreceptors located in the renal afferent arterioles is discussed in more detail later in this chapter.) Directionally, a decrease in plasma volume leads to an increase in ADH secretion and vice versa. In this pathway, afferent fibers ascend in the vagus and glossopharyngeal nerves to the nucleus tractus solitarius (NTS) and then postsynaptically project to the paraventricular and supraoptic nuclei.

Of these two control systems, the osmoreceptor pathway is almost certainly the most important for minute-to-minute control of ADH secretion. As illustrated in Fig. 5-5, very small changes in plasma osmolarity (< 1%) can lead to significant changes in ADH secretion and therefore plasma ADH concentration. In contrast, relatively large changes in blood volume and pressure of 10% or more must occur before effects on ADH secretion can be detected. These two control systems do interact, however. In particular, volume status can affect the secretory response to changes in plasma osmolarity. As illustrated in Fig. 5-6, the sensitivity of the osmoreceptor-mediated pathway increases under conditions of decreased plasma volume. In other words, for any given increase in plasma osmolarity, the amount of ADH secreted will be greater under conditions of reduced plasma volume. Note also in Fig. 5-6 that the so-called osmotic set point is affected by volume status. In this context, the set point is the osmolarity below which ADH secretion is zero. Thus, a decrease in plasma volume lowers the osmotic set point, and ADH is then released at a lower plasma osmolarity. Conversely, an increase in plasma volume above normal elevates the set point. Homeostatically, this presumably implies that under conditions of severe volume depletion, the restoration of plasma volume is a higher priority than the maintenance of plasma osmolarity.

Fig. 5-7 illustrates two important points regarding plasma ADH concentration. First, as with other endocrine systems, normal circulating levels of ADH are extremely low, typically on the order of 10^{-9}–10^{-10} M (pg/mL) or less. Second, relatively small changes in plasma ADH concentration elicit major changes in overall renal function. In the example presented, a range of ADH concentrations from 0 pg/mL to just 5 pg/mL or so dictates whether the kidneys are in a state of either maximal diuresis or maximal antidiuresis. This again implies that the sensitivity of the system is extremely high. Indeed, it has been established that a 1% change in plasma osmolarity is sufficient to change plasma AVP levels by 1 pg/mL. Functionally, a 1 pg/mL change in plasma AVP can trigger a change in urine osmolarity of 250 mOsm/L.

Changes in plasma osmolarity, which are detected by hypothalamic osmoreceptors, and changes in plasma volume, which are detected by baroreceptors, can affect ADH release.

The osmoreceptor pathway is the most important for minute-to-minute control of ADH secretion.

Changes in plasma volume affect the osmoreceptor-dependent control of ADH secretion.

Only relatively small changes in plasma ADH concentration are required to elicit major changes in overall renal function.

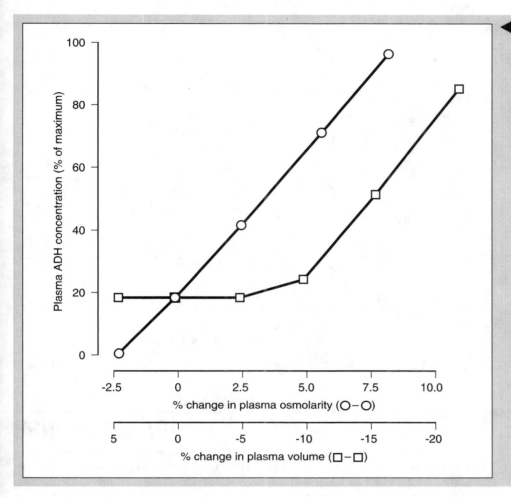

◀ *FIGURE 5-5*
*Relative Sensitivity of Osmoreceptor- ver-
sus Baroreceptor-mediated Antidiuretic
Hormone (ADH) Release.* Note that very
small changes in plasma osmolarity can
trigger large changes in ADH secretion. In
contrast, large changes in plasma volume
are required to effect ADH release. (Note
that 0 represents a normal plasma osmolarity of approximately 285 mOsm/L.)

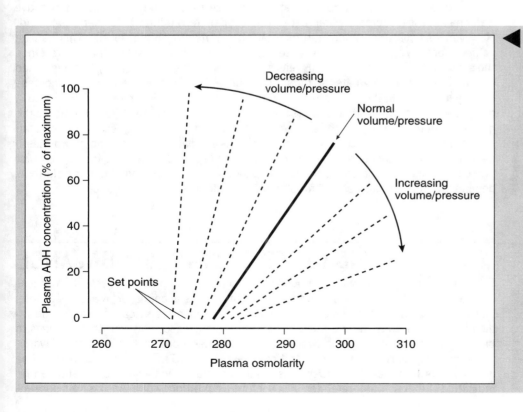

◀ *FIGURE 5-6*
*Effect of Plasma Volume Status on
Osmoreceptor-mediated Antidiuretic Hor-
mone (ADH) Release.*

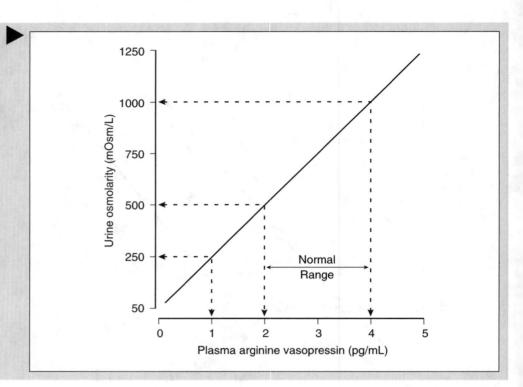

FIGURE 5-7 ▶
Relationship between Plasma Antidiuretic Hormone (ADH) Concentration and Urine Concentrating Ability. *Note that a small change in ADH concentration elicits a large change in urine osmolarity. The normal range represents typical ADH and urine osmolarity values in humans.*

THIRST RESPONSE

The preceding section emphasized the critical role that ADH plays in regulating water excretion by the kidneys. As mentioned earlier in the chapter, however, the effects of ADH alone are not sufficient to maintain total body water homeostasis. Consider a situation where there has been a net loss of total body water as a result of excessive sweating. As described above, the renal compensatory response to this state of so-called negative water balance is to increase water reabsorption and thereby minimize further loss of fluid. However, reabsorption cannot return total body water to normal levels. This can be achieved only by rapidly increasing water intake. In fact, this is exactly what occurs, since the same stimuli that regulate ADH release (increased plasma osmolarity and decreased plasma volume) also regulate the thirst mechanism. In this case, therefore, the increase in body fluid osmolarity and (depending on the severity of the water loss) the decrease in plasma volume trigger osmoreceptors and baroreceptors, respectively, and stimulate the neural centers involved in thirst (see Figs. 5-1 and 5-4). As a result, there is an increased desire to drink. Once sufficient water has been absorbed from the gastrointestinal (GI) tract to restore normal osmolarity and volume of body fluids, the increased thirst drive is terminated. Therefore, the rapid restoration of normal body fluid osmolarity is dependent on the coordinated efforts of both the kidneys and the thirst center.

The activity of the thirst center is affected by inputs from osmoreceptors and baroreceptors.

SYNDROMES OF WATER IMBALANCE

There are numerous clinical conditions that lead to the inappropriate retention or loss of total body water. Since Na+ and its attendant anions account for over 95% of total plasma osmolarity, measurement of plasma Na+ concentration can provide some indication of total body water status. It should be recognized, however, that changes in plasma Na+ concentration can occur for reasons other than a net gain or loss of water. Nevertheless, a plasma Na+ concentration of less than 135 mEq/L with a corresponding osmolarity of less than 275 mOsm/L is clinically defined as hyponatremia and can be indicative of excess water retention. Conversely, a condition with a plasma Na+ concen-

Hyponatremia is defined as a plasma Na+ concentration of less than 135 mEq/L with a corresponding osmolarity of less than 275 mOsm/L; hypernatremia is defined as a plasma Na+ concentration in excess of 145 mEq/L with an osmolarity greater than 295 mOsm/L.

tration and osmolarity in excess of 145 mEq/L and 295 mOsm/kg, respectively, is defined as hypernatremia and can be indicative of a net water deficit.

Hyponatremia

There are several possible causes of hyponatremia. Perhaps the simplest scenario is excessive fluid intake or so-called polydipsia. In this case, the degree of hyponatremia depends on the level of fluid intake relative to renal water excretion. Up to a point, the effects on plasma Na^+ concentration are minimal, since as fluid intake increases, ADH secretion and therefore water reabsorption decrease until urine output is maximal. Recall that in a human, a urine output of 18–20 L/d reflects maximal diuresis. Although somewhat unlikely, if fluid intake exceeds this maximal excretory capacity, a reduction in plasma Na^+ concentration must occur.

An alternative and more likely cause of hyponatremia can be ascribed to the dysregulation of ADH secretion. This condition, in which the normal osmoreceptor- and baroreceptor-mediated control of ADH secretion is impaired or absent, is referred to as the syndrome of inappropriate ADH secretion or SIADH. There are at least three primary causes of this syndrome. First, a persistent "leakage" of ADH can occur from the neurohypophysis, as a result, for example, of skull fractures or head trauma. Second, A resetting of the osmotic set point can occur so that the threshold for ADH release is lowered. As described earlier (see Fig. 5-6), this shift can occur simply as a result of a marked decrease in plasma volume. A similar phenomenon occurs during pregnancy. Pathophysiologically, this phenomenon also is seen with some neurologic, psychiatric, and pulmonary disorders, and sometimes as a result of drug toxicity. Finally, ADH secretion can be totally devoid of regulatory input as a result of synthesis by peripheral tumors, which have been described in numerous tissues including the lung, the GI tract, the bladder, and the prostate gland.

Additionally, there is an extensive list of pharmacologic agents that are associated with the development of hyponatremia. In some cases, these drugs enhance ADH release from the neurohypophysis. This category includes chlorpropamide, nicotine, and several narcotics. Alternatively, several drugs are thought to potentiate the renal effects of circulating ADH. This category also includes chlorpropamide as well as several nonsteroidal anti-inflammatory drugs (NSAIDs) and acetaminophen.

Hyponatremia primarily affects the central nervous system (CNS). As the plasma Na^+ concentration decreases, the osmotic flux of water into brain cells causes swelling. Up to a point, hyponatremia can be tolerated quite well by the brain, since volume regulatory mechanisms compensate for the reduction in extracellular Na^+. Below 125 mEq/L, however, the symptoms, including apathy and lethargy, nausea and vomiting, and symptoms of disorientation and confusion, become progressively more severe. Severe symptoms such as stupor, coma, or seizures can occur with profound chronic hyponatremia (serum $Na^+ < 110$ mEq/L), and in some cases, the neurologic impairment is irreversible.

SIADH occurs when normal osmoreceptor- and baroreceptor-mediated control of ADH secretion is impaired or absent.

Hypernatremia

The causes of hypernatremia are quite diverse. However, this chapter focuses on conditions in which the synthesis, secretion, or action of ADH is impaired, resulting in modest-to-profound polyuria. These conditions are collectively referred to as diabetes insipidus, meaning "large volume of tasteless fluid." (Diabetes mellitus also results in polyuria; in this case, the Latin term refers to the fact that this large volume of fluid is sweet tasting, as a result of the high concentrations of glucose.) Diabetes insipidus can be categorized either as central or nephrogenic.

Central Diabetes Insipidus. Central diabetes insipidus is due to decreased ADH release from the neurohypophysis, which may be the result of impaired synthesis in the hypothalamus, impaired transport to the neurohypophysis, or impaired storage and secretion from the neurohypophysis. Depending on the severity of the condition, overt hypernatremia can be avoided if water intake matches urine output. This can be a challenge, however, if the diabetes insipidus results in a daily urine output of 15–20 L! The condition can be treated by administration of exogenous ADH. For many years, the

Diabetes insipidus is a condition in which ADH synthesis or secretion is impaired (central diabetes insipidus) or the renal response to circulating ADH is impaired (nephrogenic diabetes insipidus).

treatment of choice was an intramuscular injection of pitressin tannate in oil, a purified extract of vasopressin from animal pituitaries. Now, the preferred treatment is to administer a vasopressin analogue, 1-desamino-8-D-arginine vasopressin (dDAVP, desmopressin) by nasal spray. This analogue has several advantages over the native extract including enhanced antidiuretic potency, a prolonged duration of action, and diminished pressor effects. It should be noted, however, that periodic exogenous ADH treatment does not lead to the generation of maximally concentrated urine, since the extended lack of ADH between treatments and the resultant polyuria depress the medullary interstitial osmotic gradient.

Nephrogenic Diabetes Insipidus. In nephrogenic diabetes insipidus, plasma ADH levels can be quite normal or even elevated; however, the hydro-osmotic response of the collecting tubule to circulating hormone is depressed. The causes of this reduced responsiveness are not yet fully established, although in some cases the evidence indicates that mutations in the ADH receptor impair binding and thus cAMP generation. More recently, there have been reports that aquaporin synthesis and the ability to translocate aquaporins to the luminal membrane may be impaired. Fortunately, in most cases reduced responsiveness to ADH is only partial, resulting in relatively mild polyuria. Since the central osmoregulatory mechanisms are intact in this situation, the thirst center is stimulated and an increased intake of water compensates for the increased output, thereby minimizing the degree of hypernatremia.

As with hyponatremia, several drugs are associated with the development of hypernatremia. Perhaps the best known is ethanol, which can directly inhibit the release of ADH from the neurohypophysis. Other drugs, such as demeclocycline, probably antagonize the renal tubular effects of ADH. Similarly, lithium, which is widely used in the treatment of affective disorders, is associated with a renal concentrating defect in perhaps 50% of the patients undergoing this treatment.

Once again, the primary consequence of hypernatremia is impaired CNS function, this time resulting from an osmotic efflux of water and thus brain cell shrinkage. With prolonged hypernatremia the brain can in fact compensate for this osmotic imbalance. Similar to the situation described for the renal medulla (see Chap. 4), brain cells can synthesize or import a series of "organic osmolytes," including amino acids, polyol sugars, and methylamines, which increase intracellular osmolarity and thereby encourage osmotic flow of water back into the cells. This long-term compensatory mechanism subsequently requires caution when attempting to correct the systemic hypernatremia, since if normal extracellular osmolarity is re-established too quickly, the excess osmolytes within the brain cells would lead to a further influx of water and thus cell swelling, as in primary hyponatremia.

FREE WATER CLEARANCE

In Chap. 4 we described the unique transport characteristics of the ascending limb of the loop of Henle, which resulted in the generation of a hypotonic tubular fluid. In the complete absence of ADH, reabsorption of water cannot occur, but continued reabsorption of sodium chloride (NaCl) in the collecting tubule dilutes this tubular fluid even further. As a result, excreted urine could have an osmolarity of only 50 mOsm/L. Compared then to the isotonic (300 mOsm/L) fluid that was filtered, under these conditions proportionally more water than solute is being excreted. In essence then the urine can be considered to be containing a volume of "solute-free" water. It should be apparent that the quantity of solute-free water that is excreted is in large part determined by the circulating levels of ADH. For example, no solute-free water is excreted when ADH-dependent reabsorption of water results in the generation of an isotonic urine. As ADH titers increase further, reabsorption of water results in the generation of hypertonic urine, at which point proportionally more solute than water is excreted.

The ability to generate, and the ultimate fate of free water can be quantified and is ultimately expressed as free water clearance. This term is somewhat deceiving since the standard clearance formula is not used to calculate this value; it is calculated as follows:

Free water clearance (C_{H_2O}) = $\dot{V}$ – C_{OSM}, where

C_{OSM} = total osmolar clearance = $\dfrac{\dot{V} \times U_{OSM}}{P_{OSM}}$ and

U_{OSM} and P_{OSM} = urine and plasma osmolarity, respectively and

$\dot{V}$ = urine flow rate

Based on the discussions above, the value for free water clearance is positive when hypotonic urine is excreted and negative when hypertonic urine is excreted. Indeed, under these latter conditions a new term is often substituted ($T^c_{H_2O}$) or free water reabsorption. Simply, free water clearance represents the amount of distilled water that must be either added to (during antidiuresis) or removed from (during diuresis) urine to create an isotonic fluid. The following examples illustrate this concept. Assume for ease of calculation that plasma osmolarity is 300 mOsm/L in all cases.

During diuresis, 5 L of 150 mOsm/L urine are excreted over a 24-hour period:

$$C_{H_2O} = \dot{V} - \frac{\dot{V} \times U_{OSM}}{P_{OSM}}$$
$$C_{H_2O} = 5000 \text{ mL} - \frac{(5000 \text{ mL} \times 150 \text{ mOsm/L})}{300 \text{ mOsm/L}}$$
$$= 5000 \text{ mL} - 2500 \text{ mL} = 2500 \text{ mL/d}$$

During antidiuresis, 750 mL of 1050 mOsm/L urine are excreted over a 24-hour period:

$$C_{H_2O} = \dot{V} - \frac{\dot{V} \times U_{OSM}}{P_{OSM}}$$
$$C_{H_2O} = 750 \text{ mL} - \frac{(750 \text{ mL} \times 1050 \text{ mOsm/L})}{300 \text{ mOsm/L}}$$
$$= 750 \text{ mL} - 2625 \text{ mL} = -1875 \text{ mL/d, or}$$

$$T^c_{H_2O} = +1875 \text{ mL/d}$$

Finally: 2 L of 300 mOsm/L urine are excreted over a 24-hour period.

$$C_{H_2O} = \dot{V} - \frac{\dot{V} \times U_{OSM}}{P_{OSM}}$$
$$C_{H_2O} = 2000 \text{ mL} - \frac{(2000 \text{ mL} \times 300 \text{ mOsm/L})}{300 \text{ mOsm/L}}$$
$$= 2000 \text{ mL} - 2000 \text{ mL} = 0 \text{ mL/d}$$

The primary diagnostic value of measuring free water clearance is that it provides a noninvasive assessment of the efficiency of transport function in the thick ascending limb. Experimentally, C_{H_2O} is measured after administration of an oral water load. The reasoning behind this is that the excess water should suppress ADH levels effectively to zero, and therefore a very dilute urine should be excreted. (In some cases ADH antagonists are also administered to ensure that residual levels of circulating ADH are ineffective.) The degree to which this urine is diluted depends primarily on the function of the thick ascending limb. In this context, then, there are a number of clinical scenarios in which thick ascending limb transport and thus free water clearance is reduced. As discussed in Chap. 4, these include adrenal insufficiency (Addison's disease) and Bartter's syndrome (although some clinical studies report no change in C_{H_2O} in this disease).

The primary diagnostic value of measuring free water clearance is the noninvasive assessment of the efficiency of transport function in the thick ascending limb.

MAINTENANCE OF BODY FLUID VOLUMES

The regulation of total body Na+ content is crucial for the maintenance of body fluid volumes. Most body Na+ is retained within the ECF compartment primarily as a result of the activity of the plasma membrane Na+–K+-ATPase, which maintains relatively low intracellular Na+ content. As a result of this distribution, any net increase in total body Na+ is retained within the ECF compartment, and volume of this fluid compartment then increases. Conversely, a net loss of total body Na+ results in a decrease in ECF volume. To illustrate this concept, consider, for example, the effects of a net gain of NaCl as a result of ingesting salt tablets (Fig. 5-8).

FIGURE 5-8 ▶

Initial Effects of a Change in Total Body Sodium Content and Activated Compensatory Mechanisms. *Note that the inverse relationship between extracellular (ECF) osmolarity and intracellular (ICF) volume implies that with, for example, an increase in ECF osmolarity, there must be an osmotic flux of water from the ICF to the ECF.*

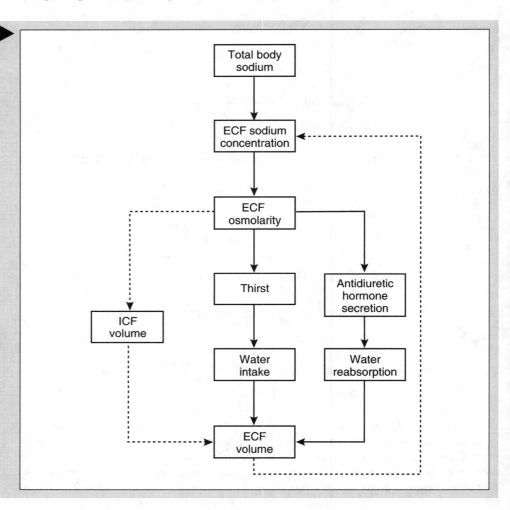

Once absorbed from the GI tract this NaCl will be almost completely retained within the ECF compartment as a result of Na+–K+-ATPase activity. It is reasonable to assume that this net gain of Na+ in the ECF leads to a sustained increase in ECF Na+ concentration. However, this does not occur. *Initially*, there is a small rise in ECF Na+ concentration and therefore ECF osmolarity. However, since the ECF is now hypertonic with respect to the ICF, water moves osmotically from the ICF to the ECF compartment until a new equilibrium osmolarity is achieved. At that point, the ECF volume is increased and the ICF is decreased. However, even after this initial osmotic shift of water has occurred, ECF osmolarity is still elevated. As discussed in the previous section, this hypertonic condition stimulates ADH secretion and therefore water reabsorption and water ingestion increase via the thirst response. This state of enhanced water conservation and intake continues until ECF osmolarity returns to normal. At this point however,

Most total body Na+ is retained within the ECF compartment as a result of the activity of Na+–K+-ATPase. Pure changes in total body Na+ can therefore affect ECF osmolarity.

ECF volume is even further expanded. Complete restoration of volume homeostasis can be achieved only after this excess load of NaCl is excreted by reducing renal tubular Na+ reabsorption. This is, at least in part, accomplished by decreasing plasma aldosterone levels.

At the other extreme, a pure loss of total body Na+ initially decreases ECF osmolarity, which causes the osmotic movement of water from ECF to ICF compartments until osmotic equilibrium is achieved. At this point, ECF volume is decreased and ICF volume is increased. Yet, ECF osmolarity is still low; therefore, ADH-dependent water reabsorption and water intake remain suppressed until normal osmolarity has been restored. Restoration of osmolarity, however, causes a further decrease in ECF volume (see Fig. 5-8). Complete restoration of volume homeostasis in this case can be achieved only when total body Na+ returns to normal levels. This is accomplished by creating a temporary situation in which dietary intake of Na+ exceeds urinary output. During this phase, renal tubular Na+ reabsorption is increased to minimize excretion. Several mechanisms, including increased plasma aldosterone levels, are involved in this process.

Two issues should be emphasized before continuing. First, the examples presented above were oversimplified for illustrative purposes. In reality, the shifts in fluid volumes and osmolarities and the changes in ADH levels occur in a continuous, dynamic fashion rather than in the deliberate, stepwise fashion presented. Second, it is important to understand that the kidneys can regulate the excretion of water and Na+ independently. In many instances, however, the challenge to overall body fluid homeostasis involves disturbances in both water and Na+ balances, and, therefore, requires coordinated responses involving both ADH and aldosterone. A common example of this is severe sweating in which there is a net loss of both salt and water as hypotonic fluid. This scenario is discussed in more detail later in this chapter.

The kidneys can regulate the excretion of water and Na+ independently.

Positive and Negative Sodium Balance

In the somewhat simplified scenario described above, we considered the effects of an acute change in total body Na+ content on body fluid homeostasis and the compensatory changes that occur. In the case of salt tablet ingestion, the increase in volume is transient, lasting only as long as it takes to excrete the excess Na+. The effects are different with a sustained change in Na+ intake. Consider what happens when dietary Na+ intake is suddenly doubled and sustained for a period of several days (Fig. 5-9). Prior to the dramatic increase in intake, Na+ excretion precisely matches Na+ intake. Ideally, the kidneys would respond immediately by increasing excretion to a level that equals the new elevated level of Na+ intake. In reality this does not occur, and it may in fact take several days for the kidneys to adapt. During this transition, therefore, Na+ intake exceeds output, and as a result there is an increase in total body Na+ content. This condition is referred to as *positive Na+ balance*. During this time, ECF volume increases, since, as described earlier, additional Na+ causes an increase in osmolarity, which in turn stimulates ADH release and causes water retention. The net increase in ECF volume is reflected in a net increase in body weight. Eventually, a new steady state is achieved (plateau phase of Fig. 5-9) in which the new level of Na+ intake is again exactly matched by an increased rate of excretion. This new expanded ECF volume will be maintained as long as Na+ intake is held at this new level. If, however, dietary intake is abruptly returned to original levels, the system must once again go through a transition phase. In this case, there will be a period of time where Na+ excretion exceeds Na+ intake. This condition, referred to as *negative Na+ balance*, will continue until intake and output of Na+ are once more in equilibrium. At this point, ECF volume and therefore body weight will have returned to the values existing before the period of increased dietary Na+ intake.

Renal compensation for abrupt sustained changes in Na+ intake takes time to develop. During this transition phase, total body Na+ content will change until a new steady state is achieved.

FIGURE 5-9 ▶

Concept of Positive and Negative Na⁺ Balance. The figure illustrates the effects of an abrupt doubling of Na⁺ intake (dotted line) on Na⁺ excretion (solid line). The increased intake is maintained for a period of 6 days and then abruptly returned to the original level.

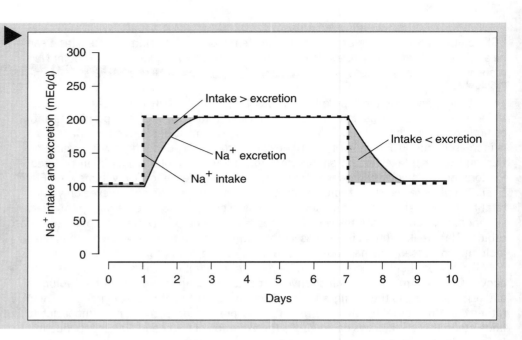

REGULATION OF ALDOSTERONE SECRETION

One of the principal factors involved in the regulation of Na⁺ excretion is the hormone aldosterone, which affects Na⁺ reabsorption in the cortical collecting tubule. One key issue to address, therefore, is how the secretion of aldosterone from the adrenal cortex is regulated. You will recall from earlier discussions that changes in plasma osmolarity detected by hypothalamic osmoreceptors were primarily responsible for the regulation of ADH secretion. One might reasonably assume that since aldosterone helps to regulate total body Na⁺ levels, there must be sensors that detect plasma Na⁺ concentration. In fact, this is probably not the case. In the simple examples described above, the ECF Na⁺ concentration changes little if at all after final compensation by the ADH system despite the net change in total body Na⁺. Similarly, there are many other scenarios where total body Na⁺ *content* may change, thus requiring an appropriate change in aldosterone secretion, but where ECF fluid Na⁺ *concentration* changes little if at all. Consider, for example, a situation where 1 L of isotonic NaCl is infused intravenously. In this case total body Na⁺ content is increased by approximately 140 mEq, but ECF NaCl concentration is unchanged since there is also a net gain of 1 L of pure water. Conversely, if 1 L of blood is withdrawn from a subject, total body Na⁺ content is decreased, but again ECF NaCl concentration remains unchanged since water is also lost. How then can changes in total body Na⁺ content be consistently detected, thereby leading to appropriate changes in aldosterone secretion? The answer is that changes in *ECF volume* primarily regulate this secretory process.

You will recall from earlier discussions that any increase in total body Na⁺ leads to an increase in ECF, while any decrease in total body Na⁺ leads to a decrease in ECF. Although changes in total ECF volume cannot be monitored, changes in plasma volume, which is one component of the ECF compartment, can indeed be accurately monitored by both the low- and high-pressure baroreceptors. Therefore, it is changes in plasma volume that lead to changes in aldosterone secretion. Many texts refer to the fact that these baroreceptors are monitoring the status of the so-called effective circulating volume or ECV, which is actually quite different from total plasma volume. In essence, this is considered to be the volume of plasma that is actually perfusing the tissues. In most cases, the ECV provides a reliable estimate of total body Na⁺. However, as we shall see later in the chapter, this monitoring system can be "tricked" into incorrectly "thinking" that total body Na⁺ has changed. For example, immersing a subject to the neck in water causes pooling of the blood in the upper torso; although total plasma volume is normal,

*Baroreceptors monitor the status of the **effective circulating volume** (or ECV), which is directly related to total body Na⁺ content.*

pooling leads to an apparent increase in ECV. This causes increased firing of the baro-receptors, which leads to a series of responses that are appropriate for a true increase in volume, including increased Na+ excretion.

RENIN–ANGIOTENSIN–ALDOSTERONE SYSTEM

In the system responsible for the regulation of ADH secretion, there is a direct neural connection between the sensors (either osmoreceptors or baroreceptors) and the supra-optic and paraventricular sites of ADH synthesis. In marked contrast, the lines of communication between the baroreceptor sensors and the ultimate release of al-dosterone from the adrenal cortex are somewhat more indirect (see Fig. 5-10). As discussed in Chap. 3, the rate-limiting step in this process is the release of the proteolytic enzyme renin from the kidney. Circulating renin, in turn, cleaves a 55–65-kD globular glycoprotein angiotensinogen, which is synthesized by and released from the liver, into the relatively inactive decapeptide angiotensin I. Subsequently, angiotensin I is further metabolized, mostly in the lungs, into the octapeptide angiotensin II by converting enzyme (dipeptidyl carboxypeptidase). Angiotensin II then directly stimulates the re-lease of aldosterone from the zona glomerulosa cells of the adrenal cortex. Most of the effects of angiotensin II, including stimulation of aldosterone secretion, are mediated by binding to AT_2 receptors, which can be blocked by the receptor antagonist losartan.

Under most circumstances, neither the availability of circulating angiotensinogen nor the activity of angiotensin-converting enzyme (ACE) is rate-limiting in this signaling cascade. It should be noted, however, that ACE inhibitors such as captopril are frequently used both clinically and experimentally to interrupt this pathway by preventing the conversion of angiotensin I to angiotensin II. In contrast, the release of renin from the kidney is under very precise control. Renin is synthesized by modified aortic smooth muscle cells, the so-called granular cells located on the afferent arteriole. These cells are included in a complex described in Chap. 3, which is known as the juxtaglomerular apparatus. This complex also includes the efferent arteriole and the macula densa cells located on the section of the cortical thick ascending limb of the loop of Henle, which passes between the afferent and efferent arterioles.

> *The release of renin from the granular cells of the juxtaglomerular apparatus is the rate-limiting step in the ultimate secretion of aldosterone from the adrenal cortex.*

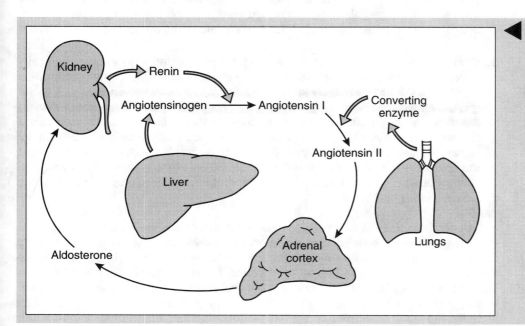

FIGURE 5-10
Renin–Angiotensin–Aldosterone System. The initial and rate-limiting step in this pathway is the release of renin from the kidney. Renin substrate (angiotensinogen) is synthesized by the liver, and most but not all angiotensin I conversion to an-giotensin II occurs in the lungs, catalyzed by angiotensin-converting enzyme.

If we consider the responses initiated in response to a drop in blood pressure and volume resulting from hemorrhage, there are at least three mechanisms that can regulate the release of renin from the granular cells (Fig. 5-11):

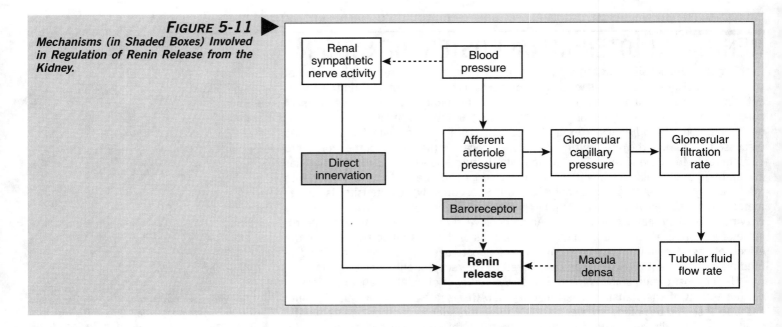

FIGURE 5-11 ▶

Mechanisms (in Shaded Boxes) Involved in Regulation of Renin Release from the Kidney.

The release of renin is controlled by three interactive mechanisms: renal barorecep- tors, renal sympathetic nerves, and the macula densa.

1. **Intrarenal baroreceptors.** The drop in blood pressure is sensed directly by the granular cells, which act as baroreceptors, and results in the increased release of renin.

2. **Sympathetic nervous system.** The granular cells are directly innervated by renal sympathetic nerve fibers. Overall sympathetic nervous system activity increases as a result of the decrease in blood pressure, which at the level of the kidney results in increased renin release. Increased renal sympathetic nerve activity also causes con- striction of the afferent arteriole (see Chap. 3). Since this occurs predominantly upstream of the granular cells, increased resistance causes a further reduction in downstream pressure resulting in further enhancement of baroreceptor-mediated renin release.

3. **Macula densa.** The reduction in blood pressure, coupled with a sympathetically driven increase in afferent arteriolar resistance leads to a drop in glomerular filtration rate (GFR). As a result, tubular fluid flow rate to the loop and more specifically to the macula densa, decreases. This decrease is sensed and results in increased renin secretion. Although still the subject of considerable debate, it is proposed that a change in Cl$^-$ delivery to and transport by the macula densa cells are the primary signals to alter renin secretion by the granular cells. Perhaps even less is known about the specific signal that connects the macula densa to the granular cells, although adenosine, Ca^{2+}, nitric oxide, and prostaglandins have all been proposed as signaling intermediaries in this pathway.

Under most circumstances, these three mechanisms operate in an interactive fash- ion to regulate renin release. It should be noted, however, that each of these regulatory systems can operate independently. One issue relating to the macula densa deserves further clarification. You will recall from Chap. 3 that the macula densa is not only involved in the regulation of renin release but that it is also a critical component of the tubuloglomerular (TG) feedback system, which plays an important role in the regulation of GFR. The basic principles of the TG feedback system would predict that in the hemorrhage model described above, the drop in blood pressure causes a drop in GFR, which in turn should lead to a macula densa–mediated dilation of the afferent arteriole to restore GFR to normal levels. In this particular case, an increase in GFR would be homeostatically inappropriate since fluid conservation is now of the highest priority because of the blood loss. In fact, the TG feedback signal will be overridden by the hemorrhage-induced increase in renal sympathetic nerve activity and increase in circulating angiotensin II, which will cause vasoconstriction of the afferent arteriole and thereby reduce GFR.

MULTIPLE EFFECTS OF ANGIOTENSIN II

There is no question that angiotensin II is the principal factor responsible for the release of aldosterone from the adrenal cortex. It would be an understatement, however, to say that this is the only physiologic role of angiotensin II. In response to hemorrhage, angiotensin II mediates multiple responses that are aimed at returning blood pressure and volume toward normal as quickly as possible (Fig. 5-12). In this context, we can subdivide these effects into relatively acute and long-term responses. The short-term effects are designed to return blood pressure toward normal despite the fact that blood volume remains markedly depressed. This can be accomplished in several ways. Recall that blood pressure is determined by both total peripheral resistance (TPR) and cardiac

> *Angiotensin II stimulates the release of aldosterone and mediates multiple responses that are aimed at returning blood pressure and volume toward normal as quickly as possible.*

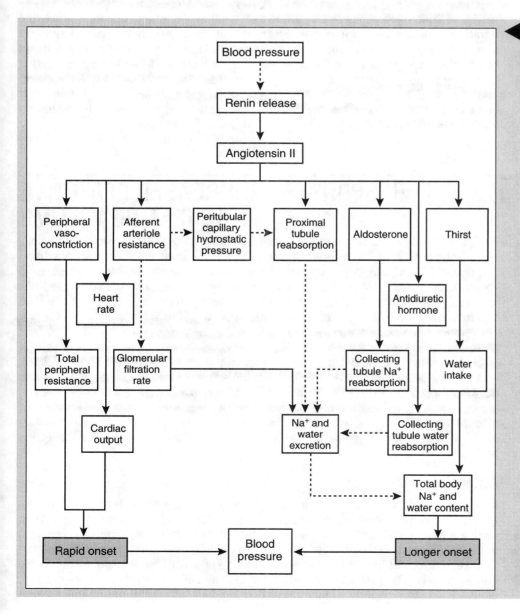

FIGURE 5-12
Multifactorial Role of Angiotensin II in Regulation of Extracellular Fluid Volume and Blood Pressure. As depicted by the shaded boxes, the effects of angiotensin II can be subdivided into either rapid-onset or longer onset responses.

output. Increased angiotensin II levels can affect both of these parameters. First, angiotensin II is a potent constrictor of vascular smooth muscle, and thus tends to increase TPR. Second, angiotensin II facilitates the effects of the sympathetic nervous system to increase cardiac output by potentiating the presynaptic release of catecholamines.

Recall that within the kidney, in addition to increasing overall TPR, the angiotensin II–mediated vasoconstriction also reduces glomerular capillary hydrostatic pressure (P_{GC}) and thus causes a drop in GFR, which in turn helps to minimize further Na^+ and water losses in the urine. In concert with the reduction of GFR described above, several other angiotensin II–mediated responses also minimize further Na^+ and water losses in the urine. For example, as described in earlier chapters, there is evidence to suggest that angiotensin II can directly increase NaCl reabsorption by the proximal tubule. In addition, as a result of differential constrictive effects on the afferent versus efferent arteriole, there is an increase in the percentage of plasma filtered (filtration fraction) that alters peritubular capillary Starling forces in such a direction as to favor proximal tubule fluid reabsorption. As discussed in Chap. 4, an increase in filtration fraction leads to an increase in efferent arteriolar protein concentration and thus an increase in peritubular capillary oncotic pressure, which alone favors increased fluid reabsorption. Additionally, however, the angiotensin II–mediated increase in afferent and efferent arteriolar resistance results in a further reduction in peritubular capillary hydrostatic pressure, a force that typically opposes fluid reabsorption. What may not be as apparent is why the filtration fraction increases in response to increased angiotensin II levels. In its simplest terms, this occurs because the reduction in renal plasma flow is proportionally much greater than the decrease in GFR. In addition to the increase in NaCl reabsorption that occurs in response to increased aldosterone levels, angiotensin II stimulates ADH release from the posterior pituitary, thereby increasing water reabsorption. Finally, angiotensin II also can act centrally to increase thirst, thereby facilitating increased water intake to help replace the losses resulting from hemorrhage.

RESPONSE TO INCREASED EFFECTIVE CIRCULATING VOLUME

To this point we have considered the renal response to an overall decrease in total body Na^+ content, and thus a decrease in the ECV. For the most part, the response to an increase in ECV will be exactly opposite. For example, the increase in blood pressure and volume suppresses renin release since (1) intrarenal baroreceptors are stimulated to a lesser degree, (2) sympathetic nervous system activity is reduced, and (3) tubular fluid flow to the macula densa is increased. This increased fluid flow is the result of an increase in GFR as well as a decrease in proximal tubular fluid reabsorption. The rise in GFR and reduced tubular reabsorption is caused by the reduction in both circulating angiotensin II levels (resulting from the decrease in renin secretion) and in sympathetic nerve activity. Additionally, the general decrease in afferent and efferent arteriolar tone also decreases the filtration fraction. This in turn leads to increased peritubular capillary hydrostatic pressure and reduced colloid osmotic pressure, thereby decreasing proximal tubule fluid reabsorption. Finally, the reduction in renin and angiotensin II decreases circulating levels of aldosterone, thereby reducing Na^+ reabsorption by the cortical collecting tubule.

Atrial Natriuretic Peptide

In addition to this series of responses, which is primarily mediated via the renin–angiotensin system, there is considerable evidence to suggest that additional factors can facilitate the excretion of NaCl and water, at least under conditions of marked expansion of the ECV. One such factor is atrial natriuretic peptide (ANP), which was first isolated from atrial myocytes in 1980 and shown to induce a powerful natriuresis when reinjected into assay rats. The precursor, pro-ANP, consists of 126 amino acids. Currently, it is believed that this peptide can be cleaved to produce at least three fragments with

Atrial natriuretic peptide (ANP) may facilitate the excretion of NaCl and water under conditions of marked expansion of the ECV.

biologic activity. This peptide elicits both renal and extrarenal effects that essentially reinforce the responses described above, as illustrated below (Fig. 5-13):

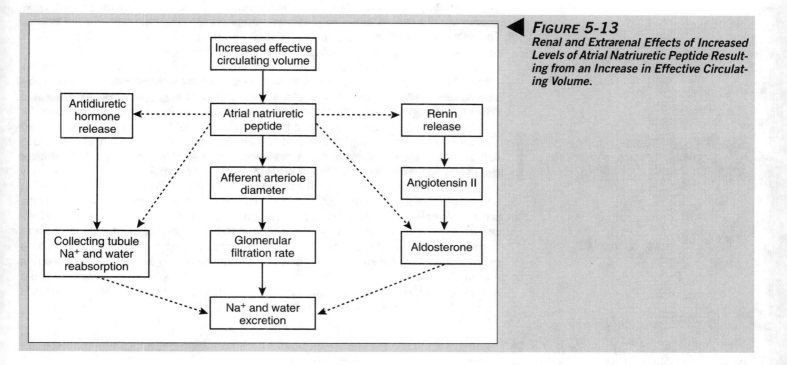

FIGURE 5-13
Renal and Extrarenal Effects of Increased Levels of Atrial Natriuretic Peptide Resulting from an Increase in Effective Circulating Volume.

1. ANP can primarily cause vasodilation of the afferent and some vasoconstriction of the efferent arterioles leading to an increase in GFR.
2. ANP can inhibit renin secretion by granular cells. This in turn reduces the levels of the vasoconstrictor angiotensin II and the levels of aldosterone. This latter effect is a result of both reduced levels of angiotensin II and a direct inhibitory effect of ANP at the level of the adrenal cortex.
3. Also, ANP can elicit a direct inhibitory effect on Na^+ reabsorption primarily in the papillary collecting tubule, probably by inhibiting the activity of the amiloride-sensitive Na^+ channel on the luminal membrane. This results from ANP binding to a so-called guanylate cyclase A (GC-A) receptor, resulting in the intracellular generation of cyclic guanosine monophosphate (cGMP). Channel block may subsequently occur as a result of both a direct effect of this cyclic nucleotide as well as via phosphorylation by cGMP-dependent protein kinase.
4. Finally, since this increase in ECV results from an excess of water as well as NaCl, ANP can also directly inhibit the release of ADH from the posterior pituitary as well as antagonize the action of ADH to increase water permeability of the collecting tubule system.

More recently, two structurally similar peptides have been identified. The first was originally discovered in the brain and thus termed brain natriuretic peptide (BNP). Significant quantities of this peptide are also found in the heart and circulatory system. Although BNP levels may be 20% that of ANP under basal conditions, plasma BNP levels can actually exceed those of ANP under certain conditions such as severe congestive heart failure (CHF). Generally, the physiologic effects of BNP are similar to those of ANP. The other structurally similar peptide occurs predominantly in the brain and has been termed CNP (simply for alphabetical consistency: **A**NP, **B**NP, **C**NP!). The specific role of this peptide has yet to be confirmed. However, since it has not been identified in plasma, the suggestion has been made that it may play an autocrine rather than endocrine role.

Putative Natriuretic Factors Synthesized Intrarenally

Under this general category of natriuretic compounds, several other factors that are synthesized by the kidney should also be considered. For example, dopamine is synthesized by proximal tubule cells and is thought to act locally to modulate Na^+ excretion. The substrate for dopamine synthesis, L-dopa, enters proximal tubule cells via a Na^+-dependent cotransporter (see Chap. 2) where it is enzymatically decarboxylated to form dopamine. Quite logically, this biosynthetic process is stimulated when animals are placed on a high-salt diet. Mechanistically, dopamine is thought to inhibit Na^+-K^+-ATPase activity in several nephron segments including the collecting tubule and thick ascending limb of the loop of Henle, resulting in reduced Na^+ reabsorption.

Several studies have established that acute intrarenal infusions of bradykinin can also elicit a natriuresis and diuresis in the absence of changes in GFR and that this results from a direct inhibition of Na^+ reabsorption in both the collecting tubule and the thick ascending limb of the loop of Henle. Similar to dopamine, bradykinin is likely generated intrarenally by the renal kallikrein–kinin system. As depicted in Fig. 5-14, tissue kallikreins, which are serine proteases, have been identified in the glomerulus, proximal tubule, and distal tubule. These enzymes convert kininogen substrate to lysine–bradykinin (kallidin), which is subsequently metabolized to bradykinin by aminopeptidase enzymes. The bradykinin in turn can be metabolized to inactive products as a result of the activity of kininases. Interestingly, kininase II is an angiotensin I–converting enzyme; hence the effects of treatment with ACE inhibitors such as captopril should always be interpreted with caution since ACE inhibitors not only suppress angiotensin II generation but also accentuate intrarenal bradykinin levels.

> Dopamine and bradykinin are two intrarenally synthesized factors that can increase Na^+ excretion.

FIGURE 5-14 ▶
Primary Components of Intrarenal Bradykinin Biosynthesis and Catabolism.

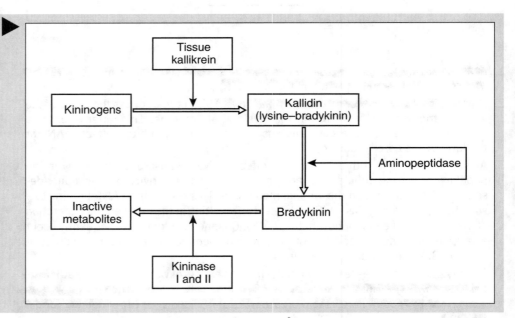

"INAPPROPRIATE" RENAL RESPONSES

Earlier in this chapter, it was emphasized that a direct relationship exists between the ECV and total body Na^+ content. Changes in ECV can be detected by a series of low- and high-pressure baroreceptors and can lead to adjustments in renal Na^+ handling to restore normal body Na^+ levels and thus restore normal ECV. There are certain circumstances, however, when this feedback mechanism is triggered "inappropriately" and thus can actually cause further deterioration in body fluid homeostasis rather than improve it. A good example of this is the development of edema. Recall from Chap. 1 that edema is a condition where there is an accumulation of excess fluid (typically > 2–3 L) within the interstitial space. The trigger for this edematous state is typically an alteration in the balance of Starling forces that are responsible for the filtration and reabsorption of fluid that occur across the capillaries.

Consider then what happens when capillary oncotic pressure is *decreased*. This can occur as a result of decreased plasma protein synthesis because of liver damage or as a result of excess protein excretion in the urine that can occur in the nephrotic syndrome. As illustrated in Fig. 5-15, a reduction in capillary oncotic pressure results in an accumulation of fluid within the interstitial space, since one of the principal driving forces for reabsorption of fluid is reduced. At this point, the accumulation of fluid within the interstitial space results in a decrease in plasma volume, or more specifically the ECV. The drop in ECV triggers the release of aldosterone via activation of the renin–angiotensin system. This, in turn, increases Na+ (and ultimately water) reabsorption and accumulation and, therefore, the size of the ECV. This causes a further reduction in plasma oncotic pressure and thus increases the net accumulation of fluid within the interstitial space. A new steady state is achieved when hydrostatic pressure within the interstitial space increases sufficiently to offset the drop in plasma oncotic pressure. In this case, then, the kidney was "tricked" into responding to a *perceived* decrease in ECF volume. In fact, in the beginning the total volume was perfectly normal, but it had been redistributed preferentially to the interstitium. The increase in Na+ and water reabsorption results in an increase in total ECF volume and exaggerates the edema.

In edema, the redistribution of fluid to the interstitial compartment results in an inappropriate Na+-retaining response as a result of a perceived decrease of ECF volume.

◄ **FIGURE 5-15**
Primary Shift in Fluid from Plasma to Interstitial Space. *This shift, such as occurs with edema, can lead to an increase in total extracellular fluid (ECF) volume.*

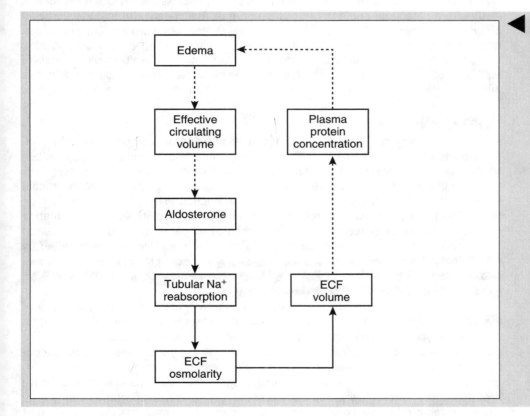

DYSREGULATION OF THE RENIN-ANGIOTENSIN-ALDOSTERONE SYSTEM

Hypoaldosteronism

The principal consequences of hypo-aldosteronism are volume depletion, hyperkalemia, and metabolic acidosis.

The primary consequences of inappropriate reductions in circulating aldosterone levels are volume depletion resulting from the inappropriate loss of Na^+ in the urine, hyperkalemia, and metabolic acidosis. Aldosterone not only stimulates Na^+ reabsorption in the cortical collecting tubule but also stimulates K^+ secretion. Consequently, lower aldosterone levels lead to reduced K^+ excretion, resulting in hyperkalemia. The cause of the metabolic acidosis is probably multifactorial. First, aldosterone stimulates hydrogen ion (H^+) secretion via activation of the H^+-ATPase located predominantly in the distal nephron. This reduced pumping capacity not only causes H^+ retention in the body, but it also reduces the ability of the kidney to generate HCO_3^-, resulting in metabolic acidosis (see Chap. 7). Second, the hyperkalemia results in an enhanced flux of K^+ into the ICF, causing a reflex efflux of H^+ from the ICF into the ECF, further supporting the acidosis.

There are at least three primary causes of hypoaldosteronism. The first lies at the level of the adrenal cortex itself. For example, in primary adrenal insufficiency, complete or partial destruction of the adrenal glands leads to impaired mineralocorticoid production. Alternatively, in congenital adrenal hyperplasia, impaired aldosterone production results from defects in one or more of the enzymes associated with mineralocorticoid biosynthesis. The second problem lies at the level of renal renin production, a condition referred to as hyporeninemic hypoaldosteronism. Finally, in pseudohypoaldosteronism, volume depletion, hyperkalemia, and metabolic acidosis exist despite elevated levels of both aldosterone and renin. In this condition, the most likely explanation is a defective mineralocorticoid receptor, resulting in impaired Na^+ reabsorption in the distal nephron.

Hyperaldosteronism

As might be expected, the primary consequences of inappropriate increases in circulating aldosterone levels are exactly the opposite of a mineralocorticoid deficit and include hypertension, hypokalemia, and metabolic alkalosis. Interestingly, however, either hypersecretion of endogenous aldosterone or administration of exogenous mineralocorticoid leads to only relatively transient Na^+ retention that is followed by a return to normal Na^+ balance within a few days. This return to normal balance despite elevated circulating mineralocorticoid is referred to as mineralocorticoid escape. Mechanistically, increased Na^+ reabsorption in the cortical collecting tubule continues. However, it is offset by decreased reabsorption in other nephron segments. For example, both increased renal arterial pressure and elevated plasma ANP levels, which result from the initial Na^+ retention, tend to decrease tubule Na^+ reabsorption.

Hyperaldosteronism can be attributed to hyperactivity of either the adrenal cortex or the renin-producing granular cells. Conn's syndrome, for example, represents a condition of primary hyperaldosteronism primarily resulting from either a benign tumor of the adrenal cortex or from bilateral adrenal hyperplasia. Primary increases in renin production can also subsequently lead to increased aldosterone production. In primary reninism, for example, tumors of the juxtaglomerular cells that secrete renin excessively have been identified. Alternatively, pathologic constriction of the renal arteries can lead to increased renin release as a result of reduced perfusion pressure across the afferent arteriole at the level of the granular cells. The consequent increases in both the vasoconstrictive actions of angiotensin II as well as the Na^+-retaining effects of aldosterone can result in so-called renovascular hypertension.

INTEGRATED RESPONSES TO CHANGES IN WATER AND SODIUM CHLORIDE BALANCE

In our earlier discussions we emphasized that the kidney has the ability to regulate the excretion of water and NaCl independently. Thus, for example, in response to a pure increase in body water content, the renal response is to increase water excretion without increasing Na+ excretion. In reality, however, many challenges to body fluid homeostasis involve perturbations in both Na+ and water balance and therefore require coordinated compensatory responses. In the case of severe hemorrhage, considered earlier in this chapter, there is a net loss of isotonic fluid. Therefore, although there is relatively little change in plasma osmolarity, the drop in ECV is sufficient to trigger the release of ADH as well as the renin–angiotensin system. But what happens in the similar but less severe situation when we donate a pint of blood. In this case, the drop in ECV is actually less than that required to stimulate ADH release but sufficient to stimulate the renin–angiotensin system. Therefore, at least in theory, ADH secretion is not increased until an aldosterone-mediated increase in Na+ reabsorption has increased plasma osmolarity. In reality, of course, the volume and Na+ are replaced quickly as a result of increased intake which is encouraged immediately after donating!

The situation differs somewhat when considering the response to severe sweating. In this case, there has been a net loss of hypotonic fluid that is a proportionally greater loss of water than Na+. The short-term consequences, therefore, are an increase in ECF osmolarity and a decrease in ECF volume. Recall, however, that the absolute drop in ECF volume as well as the absolute increase in osmolarity are partially offset by the osmotic flux of water from the ICF to the ECF. In this model, however, there are osmotic and volume stimuli for ADH release. In all of these scenarios requiring integrated responses, a key issue to consider is the time required for the ADH and aldosterone-mediated compensatory responses to take full effect. As discussed in Chap. 4, as a general rule the effects of ADH on water reabsorption occur much more rapidly than do the effects of aldosterone, primarily because the stimulatory effect of aldosterone on Na+ reabsorption requires de novo protein synthesis.

RESOLUTION OF CLINICAL CASES

Case 1

This was a patient with SIADH. Serum chemistries indicated that he was markedly hyponatremic, with a plasma Na+ concentration of 110 mEq/L compared to a normal value of 140 mEq/L. Since Na+ and its primary attendant anion Cl−, were so low, it was not surprising that serum osmolarity was also markedly reduced from a normal value of approximately 280 mOsm/L to 225 mOsm/L. The plasma creatinine concentration was relatively normal, suggesting that renal perfusion and filtration were not impaired in this patient. Under normal circumstances, one would have anticipated that a depressed serum osmolarity of this magnitude should have completely suppressed ADH secretion, resulting in the excretion of a large volume of dilute urine. In fact this was not the case, since with a volume of 500 mL over 24 hours and an osmolarity of 504 mOsm/L, there must have been a significant level of circulating ADH in this patient to have caused this degree of urine concentration. It could not be established whether or not the posterior pituitary was the source of this ADH. If so, then it would have been postulated that there was either a persistent inappropriate leakage of ADH or that the normal osmoreceptor-based control system for ADH release was impaired. However, the patient history provided no evidence of recent cranial trauma that often precipitates such events. The chest x-ray and follow-up testing indicated that this patient had a lung carcinoma, and there are many reports of such tumors being capable of synthesis and unregulated secretion of ADH. Hence, it is quite possible that this was the primary source of circulating ADH in this case. It was also quite probable that the development of this tumor may well have been smoking-related, since the patient admitted to being a heavy smoker.

It was this inappropriate retention of water that caused the considerable weight gain over the last several months. Recall that this increase in total body water adversely affects the volume and osmolarity of both the ICF as well as the ECF. In this case, dilution of the ECF caused an osmotic flux of water into the cells; hence, the volumes of the ICF and ECF were expanded, and both were at an osmolarity of 225 mOsm/L. It was the swelling of cells in the brain that most likely caused the periods of disorientation from which the patient was suffering.

Case 2

The history and present clinical symptoms are consistent with the patient suffering from CHF. The documented history of myocardial infarctions strongly suggests an impaired cardiac function probably of the left side. As a result of the inability of the left side of the heart to maintain cardiac output adequately, the blood pressure was decreased and the veins, including those in the pulmonary system, were congested leading to the shortness of breath. Not only was the venous congestion responsible for the elevated venous distention and the enlarged liver, it was also responsible for the initiation of edema formation. The increased venous pressure was reflected at the capillary level as an increase in capillary pressure resulting in the filtration of fluid from the cardiovascular system into the interstitium. It would be logical to assume that the edema was simply the result of movement of fluid from the cardiovascular system to the interstitial space. However the mechanism of the edema formation was much more complicated. The patient had gained 10 kg over the past few months, which represented a gain of 10 L of fluid. It is obvious that that much fluid cannot come solely from the cardiovascular volume, which contains only about 3 to 4 L of plasma. The ultimate source of the edema fluid was retention of Na^+ and water by the kidney. The diminished cardiac output not only resulted in a fall in blood pressure but a decreased ability to perfuse the tissues, including the kidney. The result was an increase in sympathetic nervous system drive to the kidney and, as a result, an increased renin secretion by the kidney. The resulting increase in angiotensin II, along with the increased sympathetic nervous system activity, constricted the systemic arterioles and led to increased aldosterone from the adrenal gland. The generalized vasoconstriction included the afferent arteriole in the kidney, and the GFR fell, leading to a decrease in the filtered load of Na^+. The diminished filtration rate was indicated by the increased plasma creatinine concentration found in the patient. In addition, not only was the filtered load of Na^+ and water decreased, the increased aldosterone led to an increase in Na^+ reabsorption by the kidney and subsequent Na^+ retention. It can be seen from the very low urine Na^+ concentration that the kidney was avidly retaining Na^+. The Na^+ and water were reabsorbed by the kidneys, but because of the increased systemic capillary pressure, the fluid was deposited in the interstitial space. It should be obvious that there cannot be edema without excess retention of fluid by the kidney. Because the interstitial volume is much larger than the plasma volume, the simple movement of fluid from the cardiovascular system to the interstitium would result in vascular collapse well before the volume of fluid in the interstitial space would be clinically evident. In the case presented, the plasma volume was elevated, and the veins were congested, but the effective circulating volume was decreased because of an inability of the body to perfuse the tissues adequately. It should also be intuitively obvious that loss of fluid from the cardiovascular system as a result of low colloid osmotic pressure such as occurs in the nephrotic syndrome will result in both a decrease in plasma volume and ECV. The renal response to the decreased ECV will, however, be the same in both cases, which is to conserve Na^+ and water.

REVIEW QUESTIONS

Directions: For each of the following questions, choose the **one best** answer.

1. Which combination of factors should provide the greatest stimulus for antidiuretic hormone (ADH) release?

    (A) Increased plasma osmolarity with a head-down tilt body position

    (B) Increased plasma osmolarity and a 10% loss of plasma volume

    (C) Decreased plasma osmolarity with body water immersion to the neck

    (D) Decreased plasma osmolarity and a 10% increase in plasma volume

2. Which one of the following statements is correct?

    (A) In a patient with complete hypothalamic diabetes insipidus, a single dose of exogenous antidiuretic hormone (ADH) will restore maximal concentrating ability.

    (B) A decrease in plasma volume can increase the osmotic set point for ADH release.

    (C) Fluid replacement therapy for an extended state of hypernatremia should be conducted slowly to prevent cerebral swelling.

    (D) Furosemide treatment will increase free water clearance.

3. Which one of the following statements is correct?

    (A) Hypernatremia can cause brain cell swelling.

    (B) Free water clearance is positive when antidiuretic hormone (ADH) levels are high.

    (C) Osmoreceptors can regulate both ADH secretion and the thirst center.

    (D) Both osmoreceptor- and baroreceptor-mediated increases in ADH release are associated with increased neural activity.

4. Which one of the following responses might be anticipated with a continued infusion of isotonic saline?

    (A) Increased release of aldosterone from the adrenal cortex

    (B) Increased fractional excretion of Na^+

    (C) Increased renal sympathetic nerve activity.

    (D) Decreased release of atrial natriuretic peptide (ANP) from atrial myocytes

5. Which one of the following statements concerning edema is correct?

    (A) Edema implies that there is an increased deposition of fluid in the intracellular fluid compartment.

    (B) Edema always results in a decreased plasma volume.

    (C) Edema results in a compensatory decrease in Na^+ reabsorption as a result of decreased aldosterone secretion.

    (D) Edema is initiated by an imbalance of Starling forces across the systemic capillaries.

6. Renin secretion rate by the kidney is high. Which combination of factors would decrease renin secretion most effectively?

   (A) Decreased sympathetic nervous system activity and decreased renal arterial pressure

   (B) Decreased renal arterial pressure and increased NaCl delivery to the macula densa

   (C) Increased NaCl delivery to the macula densa and decreased sympathetic nervous system activity

   (D) Increased sympathetic nervous system activity and increased renal arterial pressure

ANSWERS AND EXPLANATIONS

1. **The answer is B.** Both factors (increased osmolarity and decreased volume) stimulate the release of ADH, particularly since the decrease in plasma volume is so large. Also, the decrease in plasma volume would reduce the osmotic set point for ADH release. In option A, the increase in plasma osmolarity also stimulates ADH release; however this could be counteracted by the head-down tilt body position, which tends to pool blood in the upper torso, thereby stimulating low-pressure baroreceptors, which would suppress the release of ADH. A similar pooling of blood occurs with water immersion to the neck. In option C, this is combined with a decrease in plasma osmolarity; thus, the drive for ADH becomes essentially nonexistent. Similarly in option D, both the decrease in plasma osmolarity and the large increase in plasma volume inhibit ADH release.

2. **The answer is C.** It is now established that brain cells have the ability to synthesize "osmolytes," which offset the hypertonicity of the extracellular fluid (ECF) and thus help maintain cell volume. Once synthesized, however, if extracellular tonicity is rapidly reduced by fluid replacement, an osmotic gradient is established that drives water into those cells. Option A is incorrect, since a single dose of exogenous ADH will not restore maximal concentrating ability. This is because, as a result of the prolonged period without ADH, renal medullary osmolarity will be reduced as both NaCl and urea are washed out. With extended ADH treatment, normal medullary osmolarity and thus concentrating ability are re-established; however, this will take time. Option B is incorrect as a reduction in plasma volume in fact decreases the osmotic set point for ADH release; that is, ADH begins to be released at a *lower* plasma osmolarity. Option D is incorrect because free water is generated in the thick ascending limb of the loop of Henle as a result of selective reabsorption of NaCl without attendant water reabsorption. Since furosemide inhibits NaCl reabsorption in this nephron segment, free water clearance will decrease rather than increase.

3. **The answer is C.** An increase in plasma osmolarity leads to an increase in ADH release to conserve remaining body water and stimulates the thirst center to increase water intake, which replaces the water originally lost. Option A is incorrect because hypernatremia, which is defined as a plasma Na^+ concentration and osmolarity in excess of 145 mEq/L and 295 mOsm/kg, respectively, leads to an osmotic efflux of water from these cells, and therefore, cell shrinkage occurs. Recall, however, that depending in part on the severity of the hypernatremia, these cells can synthesize or import "organic osmolytes," which help the cells to volume regulate. Option B is incorrect, since in the presence of ADH, the free water generated in the ascending limb will be reabsorbed in the collecting tubule system. Recall that this negative free water clearance is often referred to as free water reabsorption ($T^C_{H_2O}$). Option D is incorrect because an increase in plasma osmolarity causes shrinkage of the osmoreceptor cells, leading to increased firing and increased ADH secretion. In contrast, an increase in

plasma volume increases the rate of baroreceptor firing, which in turn decreases ADH secretion.

4. **The answer is B.** Recall that the fractional excretion represents the percentage of the filtered load of Na+ that is excreted in the urine. Since continued infusion of saline tends to increase total body Na+ content, the appropriate renal response is to increase Na+ excretion. This is accomplished by increasing the glomerular filtration rate (GFR), and therefore the filtered load of Na+, and by decreasing Na+ reabsorption. In this example, the decrease in reabsorption must be greater than the increase in GFR to increase the fractional excretion. Option A is incorrect, since under these circumstances, the renin–angiotensin–aldosterone system is suppressed to reduce collecting tubule Na+ reabsorption. Conversely, depending on the extent of the volume expansion, ANP secretion is increased to facilitate Na+ excretion; therefore option D is incorrect. Finally, option C is incorrect because renal and total sympathetic nerve activity are suppressed with volume expansion.

5. **The answer is D.** Edema can occur as a result of a shift in the normal balance of Starling forces across systemic capillaries causing either an increase in filtration at the arteriolar end or a decrease in reabsorption at the venous end. Option A is incorrect since edema implies that there is a redistribution of extracellular fluid (ECF) from the plasma volume into the interstitial space. Option B is incorrect. In some edematous states, plasma volume is indeed decreased. For example, in the nephrotic syndrome, the drop in colloid osmotic pressure results in a net reduction in plasma volume. In congestive heart failure, however, plasma volume is actually increased, but impaired cardiac function results in a decrease in effective circulating volume (ECV). Option C is incorrect since the shift of fluid to the interstitial space causes a decrease in ECV, which results in increased aldosterone secretion, and thereby increased Na+ reabsorption. In fact, this is an inappropriate response, since total body Na+ content has not changed.

6. **The answer is C.** The key to the question is to remember the factors that regulate renin release: intrarenal baroreceptors are activated by a decrease in renal arterial pressure, which results in increased renin release; renin-producing granular cells are sympathetically innervated, and increased nerve activity increases renin release; and the macula densa senses some component of the delivered NaCl load, and, directionally, a decreased delivery results in increased renin secretion. In all options except C, at least one factor actually stimulates renin secretion. In option C, both the increased NaCl delivery to the macula densa as well as the decrease in sympathetic nerve activity oppose renin release.

6

MAINTENANCE OF POTASSIUM, CALCIUM, AND PHOSPHATE BALANCE

CHAPTER OUTLINE

INTRODUCTION TO CLINICAL CASES

Case 1

A 55-year-old woman has had diabetes mellitus for more than 10 years. She visited her physician every 2 months, and the disease remained in good control as a result of moderate dietary measures and the use of an oral hypoglycemic drug. Three days before admission, the patient developed a rather severe cold with mild fever. She lost her appetite and noted more frequent voiding especially during the night. A physical examination on admission revealed an acutely ill woman. Her mucous membranes were dry, and her neck veins were flat. Arterial blood pressure was 120/95 mm Hg recumbent and 90/60 mm Hg standing. Heart rate was 140 beats/min, and respiratory rate was 24 breaths/min. Urine was collected for 1 hour, and the volume was 250 mL. Laboratory values from a plasma sample were as follows: sodium (Na^+), 132 mEq/L; chloride (Cl^-), 90 mEq/L; potassium (K^+), 5.5 mEq/L; glucose, 750 mg/dL; creatinine, 2 mg/dL; and blood urea nitrogen (BUN), 40 mg/dL. A urine sample gave the following results: glucose, 4+; ketones, negative; K^+, 30 mEq/L; Na^+, 25 mEq/L; and osmolarity, 305 mOsm/L.

Case 2

A 45-year-old man was admitted to a walk-in clinic complaining of day-old severe pain in the left area of the lower back that radiated to the scrotum. He also complained of recent joint pain and weakness. His blood pressure and heart rate were 130/92 mm Hg and 90 beats/min, respectively. A routine venous blood sample resulted in the following plasma concentrations: creatinine, 1.4 mg/dL; BUN, 25 mg/dL; glucose, 82 mg/dL; Na^+, 139 mEq/L; K^+, 4.3 mEq/L; Cl^-, 101 mEq/L; and bicarbonate (HCO_3^-), 20 mEq/L. Additional plasma analysis yielded an ionized plasma calcium (Ca^{2+}) concentration of 3.2 mEq/L (high) and a total phosphorus of 1.2 mg/dL (low).

DISTRIBUTION OF TOTAL BODY POTASSIUM

An increase in extracellular K^+ concentration reduces (depolarizes) the resting membrane potential, while a decrease in extracellular K^+ concentration increases (hyperpolarizes) the resting membrane potential.

In Chap. 5 we emphasized that most total body Na^+ is confined to the *extracellular fluid* (*ECF*) compartment, primarily as a result of the activity of the cell membrane Na^+-K^+-ATPase. The activity of this pump is also responsible for the fact that most total body K^+ ($\approx 98\%$) is confined to the *intracellular fluid* (*ICF*) compartment. On a concentration basis, intracellular K^+ is approximately 120–150 mEq/L, while extracellular K^+ concentration is typically maintained at about 4 mEq/L. As the primary intracellular cation, K^+ plays an important role in cell growth and division, in the regulation of enzyme activity, and in volume regulation. The considerable concentration difference between intracellular and extracellular K^+ is also essential to the maintenance of the membrane potential. Changes in extracellular K^+ concentration can therefore have particularly adverse effects on electrically excitable tissues such as the heart and nervous system. For example, using the Nernst equation ($E_m = -61 \log([K^+]_{ICF}/[K^+]_{ECF})$, one can calculate that an increase in extracellular K^+ concentration *reduces* the resting membrane potential (depolarizes), thereby making the cell more excitable (Fig. 6-1). In contrast, a decrease in extracellular K^+ concentration *increases* the resting membrane potential (hyperpolarizes) and therefore tends to reduce the excitability of the cell (see Fig. 6-1). In general, both increases and decreases in plasma K^+ concentration can have adverse effects on neuromuscular activity, can suppress intestinal motility, and can cause ventricular arrhythmias. Clinically, a subject with an extracellular K^+ concentration of less than 3.5 mEq/L is referred to as *hypokalemic*, while a subject with an extracellular K^+ concentration of more than 5.0 mEq/L is referred to as *hyperkalemic*.

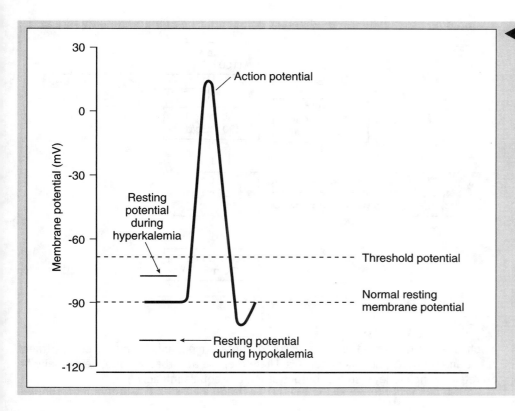

FIGURE 6-1
Effect of Extracellular Fluid (ECF) K⁺ Concentration on Resting Membrane Potential. *Using the Nernst equation, we can calculate that an increase in ECF K⁺ concentration (hyperkalemia) reduces (depolarizes) the membrane potential. In the case of electrically excitable tissues, this brings the resting potential closer to the threshold potential, thereby facilitating the generation of action potentials. In contrast, a decrease in ECF K⁺ concentration (hypokalemia) increases (hyperpolarizes) the membrane potential and therefore moves the resting potential further away from the threshold potential.*

MAINTENANCE OF PLASMA POTASSIUM CONCENTRATION

Just as we discussed for water and Na⁺, the ability to maintain a stable plasma K⁺ concentration is dependent on matching K⁺ excretion to K⁺ intake. However, the fact that plasma K⁺ concentration is so low poses an additional challenge to the maintenance of K⁺ homeostasis. Recall from Chap. 1 that total ECF volume in the prototypic human is approximately 14 L. Therefore, the total amount of K⁺ contained within the ECF is 14 L × 4 mEq/L or 56 mEq. In Western society, a typical daily diet may contain 100 mEq of K⁺, 90% of which is absorbed into the body. Since this absorbed K⁺ initially enters the ECF space, total K⁺ content and therefore concentration could theoretically almost triple (56 + 90 = 146 mEq ÷ 14 L = 10.4 mEq/L). Clearly, this does not occur, since a plasma K⁺ concentration of 10 mEq/L would be lethal. How is this avoided? It would be reasonable to assume that this excess K⁺ is simply excreted in the urine. The fact of the matter is that the absorptive process in the gastrointestinal (GI) tract adds K⁺ to the ECF faster than the kidneys can excrete it. Therefore, if no other compensation took place, there would be an inevitable marked rise in plasma K⁺ concentration. In fact, additional compensation does occur, since most of the absorbed K⁺ is initially taken up into the much larger intracellular pool and then is excreted by the kidneys over a more extended period (Fig. 6-2).

This rapid cellular uptake of K⁺ is stimulated by insulin and probably long-term by aldosterone. Mechanistically, these hormones increase the activity of the Na⁺–K⁺-ATPase, particularly in muscle, liver, and adipose tissue. The principal stimulus for increased aldosterone release is a rise in plasma K⁺. There is also evidence to suggest that insulin release is K⁺-sensitive. However, it is most likely that since plasma K⁺ is increasing during the so-called absorptive phase of the digestive process, the primary stimulus for insulin release is the absorption of glucose and amino acids. In this pathway, the absorptive process leads to the release of glucose-dependent insulinotropic peptide (GIP) from the duodenum and proximal jejunum, which in turn stimulates insulin release from the pancreas. Therefore, insulin has an effect on cellular K⁺ uptake in addition to the critical function of this hormone in regulating intermediary metabolism. It must be

> *Most of the K⁺ absorbed from the GI tract is initially rapidly taken up into the intracellular pool to prevent abrupt increases in plasma K⁺ concentration.*

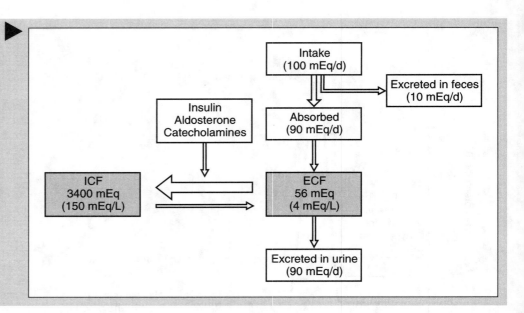

emphasized that despite the efficiency of this uptake mechanism, the ICF compartment is not an infinite-capacity sink for K+. Therefore, the absorbed K+ must eventually be excreted by the kidneys, so that output ultimately equals intake.

CHALLENGES TO POTASSIUM HOMEOSTASIS

The high intracellular K+ concentration can pose a threat to the maintenance of ECF K+ homeostasis.

The very fact that intracellular K+ concentration is so high poses a potential threat to the maintenance of a low plasma K+ concentration. In this context, there are at least four situations where this normal balance is disturbed: (1) increased plasma osmolarity, (2) cell lysis, (3) exercise, and (4) acid–base status.

Plasma Osmolarity

In previous chapters, we have emphasized that a change in plasma (ECF) osmolarity induces an osmotic flux of water across the cell membrane, thereby altering the volume of the intracellular compartment. If, for example, plasma osmolarity is increased, water will flux out of the cells, thereby reducing intracellular volume. The reduction in intracellular volume effectively increases the intracellular concentration of K+ (Fig. 6-3). As a result there will be an increased concentration gradient for K+ to flux out of the cell, which in turn increases extracellular K+ concentration.

This situation occurs in diabetes mellitus. In the absence of insulin, plasma glucose concentrations are very high. As a result, plasma osmolarity is much higher than normal, which causes an osmotic efflux of water from the intracellular compartment. This can lead to hyperkalemia due to the efflux of K+ from the cells. The absence of, or reduced responsiveness to, insulin does in fact have additional implications for K+ homeostasis; it impairs the uptake of K+ into intracellular stores during the absorptive phase of digestion. At the other extreme, administration of insulin for severe hyperkalemia is one form of treatment used to promote the cellular uptake of K+. In this case, glucose is administered along with the insulin to prevent hypoglycemia.

Cell Lysis

This is perhaps the most obvious threat to extracellular K+ homeostasis. Any time a significant number of cells are disrupted, their internal store of K+ is distributed into the ECF (Fig. 6-3). For example, hemolysis represents a condition where red blood cells (RBCs) break down, while rhabdomyolysis is a condition where skeletal muscle cells

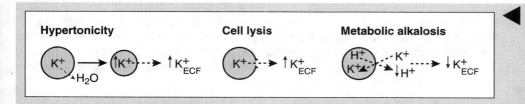

FIGURE 6-3
Three Challenges to Extracellular Fluid (ECF) K+ Homeostasis. *Hypertonicity-induced cell shrinkage effectively raises intracellular K+ concentration, leading to an increased efflux of K+ and thus an increase in ECF K+ concentration. Breakdown of the plasma membrane causes spillage of intracellular K+ into the ECF. The reduced ECF H+ concentration in metabolic alkalosis results in a primary shift of H+ out of the intracellular fluid (ICF) compartment and a reciprocal shift of K+ into the ICF. Consequently, ECF K+ concentration falls.*

break down. Similarly, a rise in plasma K+ concentration may occur during chemotherapy, when tumor cells are destroyed.

Exercise

Significant K+ efflux from skeletal muscle cells can occur during sustained exercise. This results primarily from the increased K+ efflux that is required to promote repolarization of the plasma membrane. Changes in plasma K+ concentration are relatively small (< 1 mEq/L) during mild-to-moderate exercise, however. This is due in part to the offsetting effects of catecholamines, which are typically elevated during exercise, and which can increase Na^+-K^+-ATPase activity. This effect is mediated via β_2-adrenergic receptors and results in increased cellular K+ uptake. However, during severe periods of exercise that bring a person close to the point of exhaustion, plasma K+ levels can rise as much as 2 mEq/L. Even moderate exercise may lead to greater increases in plasma K+ concentration, if the individual happens to be taking β-adrenergic blockers.

Hypertonicity, cell lysis, and exercise can cause hyperkalemia as a result of enhanced flux of K+ from ICF to ECF.

Acid–Base Status

In general terms, metabolic alkalosis can cause hypokalemia, and metabolic acidosis can cause hyperkalemia. The specific mechanisms underlying these interactions have yet to be fully understood. However, in metabolic alkalosis, it is proposed that reduced ECF hydrogen ion (H+) concentration promotes an efflux of H+ from the ICF. To maintain electrical balance across the membrane, there is a reciprocal flux of K+ from the ECF to the ICF, thereby reducing ECF K+ concentration (see Fig. 6-3). A similar rationale can be proposed for the effects of metabolic acidosis; however, the end result is dependent on whether an inorganic or organic acid is responsible for the drop in ECF pH. Overall, inorganic acids cause a more pronounced hyperkalemia. The reasoning here is that the cell membrane is relatively impermeable to the anions associated with inorganic acids, such as Cl− and sulfate; therefore, without an attendant anion, the increased flux of H+ into the ICF compartment is not electroneutral. Consequently, a reciprocal efflux of K+ must occur to maintain charge balance. In the case of organic acids, however, the attendant anions (lactate, β-hydroxybutyrate) typically have a relatively high membrane permeability. If both H+ and an attendant anion enter the cell, no reciprocal efflux of K+ is required to maintain charge balance. With similar reasoning, neither respiratory acidosis or alkalosis have significant effects on ECF K+ homeostasis, since the major contributors to this system, carbon dioxide (CO_2) and water, are freely membrane permeable.

In many cases, a primary change in ECF pH causes a reciprocal change in ECF K+ concentration.

RENAL TUBULAR TRANSPORT OF POTASSIUM

One consequence of a low plasma K+ concentration is the extremely low filtered load of K+ (4 mEq/L × 180 L/d = 720 mEq/d), compared, for example, to Na+ (140 mEq/L × 180 L/d = 25,200 mEq/d). Fig. 6-4 illustrates the fate of the filtered K+. Consistent with many other filtered solutes, approximately 65% of the filtered K+ is reabsorbed in the proximal tubule. Although still the subject of intense investigation, it is thought that only 20% or so of this K+ is reabsorbed transcellularly, while the remainder is reabsorbed paracellularly as a result of bulk flow with water. The transcellular pathway likely involves K+-selective channels on the luminal membrane.

FIGURE 6-4 ▶

Principal Renal Tubular Sites of K+ Trans-port. *Most filtered K+ is reabsorbed from the proximal tubule and the thick ascending limb, although the later sections of the collecting tubule are also capable of some reabsorption. The late distal and cortical collecting tubules are the principal sites of variable K+ secretion. Percentages represent the fraction of the filtered load of K+ transported in any given tubular segment.*

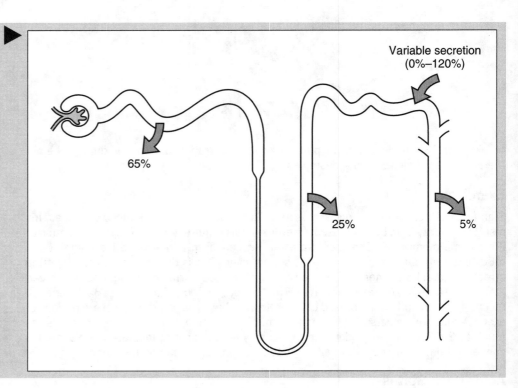

Variable secretion (0%–120%)

65%

25%

5%

Most of the filtered load of K+ that is reabsorbed in the proximal tubule and thick ascending limb occurs via the paracellular route.

An additional 25% of the filtered load of K+ is reabsorbed by the thick ascending limb of the loop of Henle. Once again, 20% or so of this K+ is reabsorbed transcellularly and 80% paracellularly. You recall from Chap. 4 that K+ enters the cell across the luminal membrane via the Na+–K+–2Cl−-cotransporter. A percentage of this entering K+ undergoes net reabsorption as a result of transport out of the cell via basolateral membrane channels and K+–Cl−-cotransporters. Most of the K+, however, refluxes into the lumen via K+ channels, thereby generating a lumen-positive potential, which is the primary driving force for the paracellular reabsorption of several cations, including K+.

Similar to renal tubular handling of Na+, approximately 10% of the filtered load of K+ is delivered to the distal nephron. Remarkably, in sharp contrast to Na+, the amount of K+ ultimately excreted in the urine usually exceeds the amount delivered to this point along the nephron. In fact, under certain circumstances, the amount of K+ excreted actually exceeds the filtered load! This is possible because the principal cells of the cortical collecting tubule are capable of *secreting* K+ into the tubular lumen. Fig. 6-5 illustrates the mechanism involved in this secretory process. Notice that it is fundamentally very similar to the mechanism responsible for Na+ reabsorption in this segment. The basolateral Na+–K+-ATPase in this case is responsible for maintaining a high intracellular K+ concentration, which provides the primary driving force for the chemically favorable movement of K+ across the luminal membrane primarily via K+-selective channels, and via a K+–Cl−-cotransporter. In addition, the reabsorption of Na+ in this nephron segment generates a lumen-negative potential, which creates a favorable electrical gradient for the movement of K+ from the cell into the lumen.

The late distal tubule cells and principal cells of the cortical collecting tubule secrete K+ into the tubular lumen.

Under normal dietary conditions, the kidney typically excretes an amount of K+ that is equivalent to approximately 20% of the filtered load. Since only 10% of the filtered load is delivered to the distal nephron, secretion into the tubular lumen must occur at the level of the collecting tubule. Under conditions of K+ deficit, tubular secretion effectively

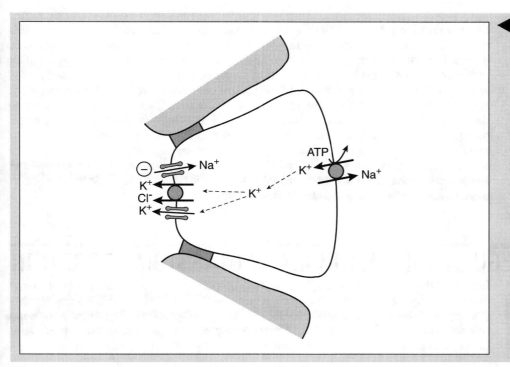

FIGURE 6-5
Mechanism of K+ Secretion by Late Distal and Cortical Collecting Tubule Cells. *K+ is transported across the luminal membrane via either K+-selective channels or via a K+–Cl−-cotransporter. Both processes depend on a favorable electrochemical diffusion gradient that is created by the high intracellular K+ concentration and the lumen-negative potential.*

stops, and there is further net reabsorption of K+ along the later sections of the collecting tubule, thereby reducing K+ excretion to 1%–2% of the filtered load. This relatively low-capacity reabsorptive mechanism is localized to the intercalated cells of the collecting tubules (Fig. 6-6). Note that the initial step of transporting K+ into the cell across the luminal membrane is mediated by an energy-dependent K+–H+-antiporter. Efflux across the basolateral membrane occurs predominantly via K+-selective channels.

As alluded to earlier, under conditions of K+ excess, K+ excretion may reach levels that are equal to or greater than the filtered load. Suppose that plasma K+ concentration

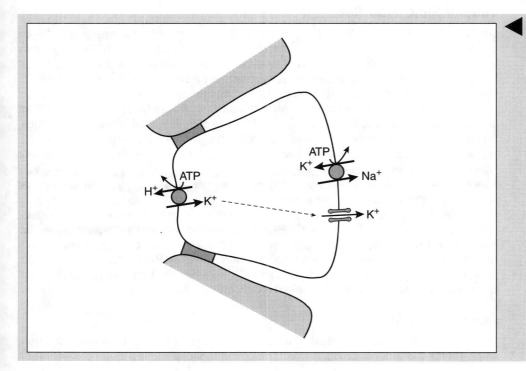

FIGURE 6-6
Mechanism of K+ Reabsorption by Inter-calated Collecting Tubule Cells. *K+ is transported across the luminal membrane into the cell by an adenosine triphosphate (ATP)–dependent K+–H+-antiporter and exits the cell across the basolateral membrane via K+-selective channels.*

has increased to 6 mEq/L. The daily filtered load would be 180 L/d × 6 mEq/L = 1080 mEq/d. Given the homeostatic need to increase K+ excretion under these circumstances, it would be reasonable to expect significant reductions in proximal tubule or thick ascending limb K+ reabsorption. In fact, this does not appear to happen. Consequently, approximately 10% of the filtered load, or 108 mEq/d, is delivered to the distal nephron. However, the amount of K+ excreted could be greater than the filtered load under these conditions, for instance 1200 mEq/d. Since only 108 mEq is delivered to the distal nephron, this suggests that a quite amazing 1092 mEq/d of K+ (1200 mEq − 108 mEq) must be secreted by the late distal and cortical collecting tubules! Clearly, this quantity of excreted K+ is not derived exclusively from the ECF compartment. Rather, most of this K+ fluxes into the ECF from intracellular stores, emphasizing that the enhanced secretion is intended to reduce total body K+ content.

REGULATION OF TUBULAR POTASSIUM SECRETION

The rate of K+ excretion is primarily determined by the rate of K+ secretion into the cortical collecting tubule; as plasma K+ concentration increases, the rate of secretion increases.

Based on the above discussion, it is evident that the rate of K+ *excretion* is primarily determined by the rate of K+ secretion. In turn, the rate of K+ *secretion* is fundamentally dependent on the magnitude of the electrochemical gradient for K+ diffusion between the intracellular environment of the collecting tubule cell and the tubular fluid. Several factors can affect this gradient and, thereby, ultimately affect K+ excretion.

Plasma Potassium Concentration

The rate of K+ secretion is fundamentally dependent on the magnitude of the electrochemical gradient for K+ diffusion between the intracellular environment of the collecting tubule cell and the tubular fluid.

Directionally, the rate of K+ secretion increases as plasma K+ concentration increases. This occurs for two major reasons (Fig. 6-7). First, the activity of the basolateral membrane Na+−K+-ATPase is directly affected by extracellular K+ levels. Second, an increase in plasma K+ directly stimulates aldosterone release from the adrenal cortex, which, in turn, increases Na+−K+-ATPase activity in the collecting tubule. As a result of this enhanced pumping capacity, intracellular K+ concentration increases, thereby enhancing the intracellular-luminal gradient for diffusion. To promote this net flux of K+ further, there is evidence to suggest that aldosterone also increases the number of K+ channels in the luminal membrane.

Tubular Fluid Flow Rate

Just as increasing intracellular K+ can enhance the transluminal membrane diffusion gradient, so too can reducing the concentration of K+ within the lumen. This is exactly what occurs when tubular fluid flow rate increases. In this case, as K+ enters the lumen, it is immediately carried downstream, thereby maintaining a lower local K+ concentration in the tubular fluid at the level of the cortical collecting tubule. This is one of several reasons why diuretic therapy can lead to K+ depletion (Fig. 6-8). Recall that diuretics block Na+ and ultimately water reabsorption, which, in the case of proximal tubule or loop diuretics, results in an increased distal tubular fluid flow rate. As a result, collecting tubule K+ secretion and thus excretion are increased. Two additional factors should be taken into consideration. First, the proximal tubule and thick ascending limb are two of the primary sites of K+ reabsorption; hence, any reduction in reabsorptive capacity in these segments reduces K+ reabsorption. In other words, more K+ is delivered to the distal nephron under these conditions. Second, if more Na+ is delivered to the cortical collecting tubule as a result of the upstream diuretic, Na+ reabsorption at this site is increased. This also increases K+ secretion, since the increased entry of Na+ into the cell across the luminal membrane (1) stimulates basolateral membrane Na+−K+-ATPase activity and therefore increases intracellular K+ concentration and (2) increases the lumen-negative potential thereby increasing the electrical gradient for K+ efflux across this membrane.

Acid−Base Status

In general terms, metabolic alkalosis increases K+ secretion and therefore excretion, while metabolic acidosis reduces secretion. Metabolic alkalosis enhances secretion

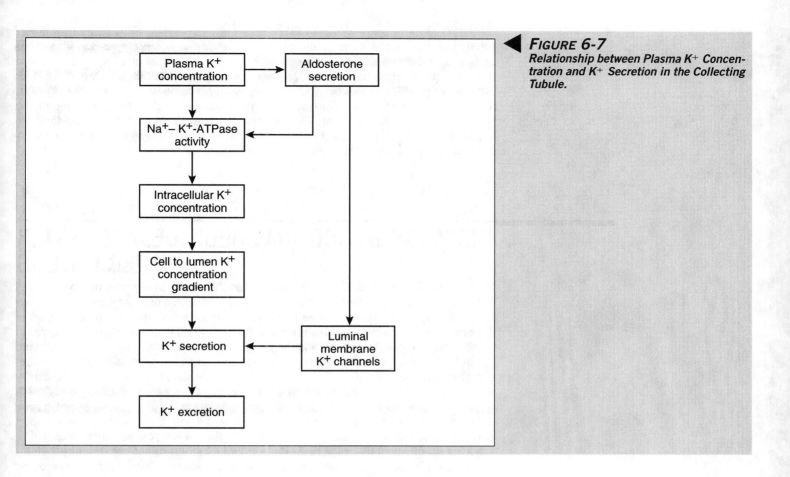

FIGURE 6-7
Relationship between Plasma K+ Concentration and K+ Secretion in the Collecting Tubule.

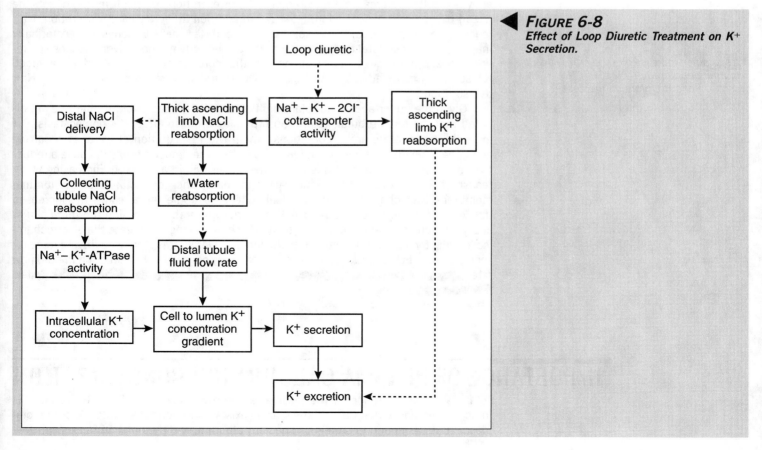

FIGURE 6-8
Effect of Loop Diuretic Treatment on K+ Secretion.

through several mechanisms. In most cells of the body, alkalosis causes an efflux of H+ and a reciprocal uptake of K+ from the ECF. This net accumulation of K+ also occurs in the cortical collecting tubule cells. Increased intracellular K+ concentration is further enhanced by a direct effect of alkalosis to increase the activity of the Na+−K+-ATPase. Additionally, alkalosis may increase both the number as well as the open time of the luminal membrane K+ channels. For the most part, the effects of metabolic acidosis are opposite to those of alkalosis; however, the effects are more pronounced under conditions of acute as opposed to chronic metabolic acidosis.

POTASSIUM, SODIUM CHLORIDE, AND WATER INTERACTIONS

In Chap. 5, we emphasized that the kidney has the ability to regulate the excretion of water and Na+ independently. For example, in response to a pure increase in total body Na+ content, the renal response is to increase Na+ excretion *without* increasing water excretion. The relationship between K+ and Na+ excretion is a little different. You recall that the cortical collecting tubule is the primary site for K+ secretion as well as a major site of Na+ reabsorption. Mechanistically, these two transport processes share a number of features, perhaps the most important of which is absolute dependence on the activity of basolateral membrane Na+−K+-ATPase. Any factor, for example, that increases the activity of this enzyme in the cortical collecting tubule should increase K+ secretion *and* increase Na+ reabsorption. The question, however, is whether both changes in transport were homeostatically necessary. For example, if plasma K+ concentration rises, Na+− K+-ATPase activity in the collecting tubule increases as a result of both the direct effect of elevated plasma K+ and the effect of elevated aldosterone levels. Increased enzyme activity results in increased K+ secretion and thus excretion, which ultimately offsets the rise in plasma K+ concentration. However, in addition to increasing K+ secretion, Na+ reabsorption is increased. In this setting, enhanced Na+ reabsorption is homeostatically inappropriate since total body Na+ content was perfectly normal. Given the close coupling between these two transport processes, therefore, an extended period of enhanced K+ secretion can lead to an increase in ECF volume as a result of inappropriate Na+ reabsorption.

> A sustained increase in K+ secretion leads to an inappropriate increase in Na+ reabsorption and therefore an increase in ECF volume.

Given the importance of tubular fluid flow rate for K+ secretion, it might be anticipated that the renal tubular water reabsorption could also affect K+ homeostasis. For example, under antidiuretic conditions, when avid reabsorption of water is occurring along the collecting tubule, one might predict that the reduced flow will cause a reduction in K+ secretion. In fact this is not the case, since in addition to increasing water reabsorption, antidiuretic hormone (ADH) increases the conductance of the luminal membrane Na+ channels in the cortical collecting tubule. As a result, the increased uptake of Na+ increases Na+−K+-ATPase activity, thereby increasing the intracellular accumulation of K+ and lumen negativity. These two changes increase the electrochemical driving force for K+ secretion into the lumen. Overall, this increased driving force for secretion offsets the reduction in secretory capacity caused by the reduction in fluid flow rate. The net result is that ADH-dependent changes in water excretion have very little impact on K+ excretion.

IMPORTANCE OF PLASMA CALCIUM ION CONCENTRATION

Total Ca2+ concentration in the plasma is approximately 4.8 mEq/L. However, it is important to realize that Ca2+ in the plasma exists in two forms. About 50% of the total plasma Ca2+ is bound to proteins, especially albumin, and the other 50% exists as free

Ca^{2+}. Free Ca^{2+} concentration in the interstitial fluid is essentially equal to that in the plasma. However, *total* Ca^{2+} concentration is considerably lower, since, relative to plasma, the interstitial fluid contains a much lower protein concentration, and thus relatively little Ca^{2+} is bound in this fluid compartment. Ultimately, it is this pool of free Ca^{2+} that is physiologically regulated. Among other things, the Ca^{2+} concentration in the interstitial fluid that bathes the cells is responsible for membrane stability. A low free Ca^{2+} concentration increases membrane excitability of nerves and muscles and may lead to hypocalcemic tetany resulting from spontaneous action potentials. On the other hand, an increase in free Ca^{2+} concentration decreases membrane excitability and can result in cardiac arrhythmias. Ca^{2+} is also involved in normal cardiac muscle contraction, in the release of some hormones, and is the major component of bone.

Relative to extracellular Ca^{2+} concentration, intracellular free Ca^{2+} concentration is very low: about 100 nEq/L compared to 2.4 mEq/L in the ECF. This large concentration difference is maintained by several mechanisms including cellular efflux via a plasma membrane Ca^{2+}-ATPase and Na^+–Ca^{2+} exchanger, as well as uptake into intracellular organelles such as the endoplasmic reticulum and mitochondria. Many intracellular events such as intracellular signaling and excitation–contraction coupling depend on transient changes in intracellular Ca^{2+} concentration.

> Plasma ionized Ca^{2+}, not total plasma Ca^{2+}, is physiologically regulated.

REGULATION OF PLASMA CALCIUM ION CONCENTRATION

Regulation of plasma Ca^{2+} concentration is dependent on the integrated function of a number of organ systems in the body, including the kidney, the GI tract, and the bones (Fig. 6-9). The plasma concentration of Ca^{2+} is determined both by uptake of Ca^{2+} from the GI tract and by the renal excretion of Ca^{2+}. Both processes are under hormonal control. Unlike most electrolytes such as Na^+ and K^+, which are almost completely absorbed, the intestinal absorption of Ca^{2+} is controlled by 1,25-dihydroxyvitamin D_3. Similarly, renal reabsorption of Ca^{2+} is controlled by parathyroid hormone (PTH). Thus, total body Ca^{2+} is determined by the regulation of both input and output.

A typical diet contains about 1 g of calcium. Approximately 20% of the ingested calcium is absorbed in the intestines, and the remainder is excreted in the stool. There is secretion of Ca^{2+} into the intestinal lumen, but the magnitude of the absorption is

> Intestinal Ca^{2+} absorption and renal excretion of Ca^{2+} are both regulated. Net Ca^{2+} balance is the difference between the two.

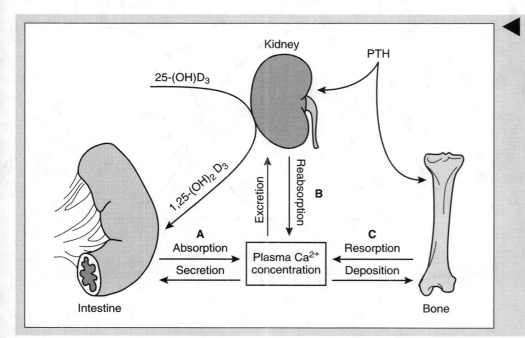

FIGURE 6-9
Interrelationship of Organ Systems Involved in Regulation of Plasma Ca^{2+} Concentration. Ca^{2+} is (A) absorbed and secreted by the intestine, (B) reabsorbed and excreted by the kidney, and (C) deposited on or resorbed from bone. Parathyroid hormone (PTH) stimulates Ca^{2+} reabsorption by the kidney and resorption from bone. 1,25-Dihydroxyvitamin D_3 (1,25-$(OH)_2D_3$) stimulates Ca^{2+} absorption by the intestine.

greater than secretion; thus, there is net uptake. The secretory rate appears to be relatively constant, but the absorptive rate can be regulated by 1,25-dihydroxyvitamin D_3. The kidney excretes approximately 1% of the filtered load of Ca^{2+}. Thus, the body has a large capacity to increase both intestinal absorption and renal excretion. The bones, which are composed mainly of the mineral $CaHPO_4$ are also involved in overall Ca^{2+} homeostasis. PTH can increase the plasma Ca^{2+} concentration by increasing the resorption of both Ca^{2+} and HPO_4^{2-} from the bone. Conversely, a decrease in plasma PTH can lead to a decrease in plasma Ca^{2+} concentration by promoting the deposition of Ca^{2+} and HPO_4^{2-} onto the bone. In the overall scheme, the most important factor in the regulation of plasma Ca^{2+} is the plasma concentration of PTH.

REGULATION OF PARATHYROID HORMONE SECRETION

Parathyroid gland secretion of PTH is stimulated by low plasma Ca^{2+} concentration and depressed by high plasma Ca^{2+} concentration.

The major regulator of plasma PTH concentration is plasma Ca^{2+} concentration. The human typically has about four parathyroid glands located in the body of the thyroid gland which synthesize, degrade, and secrete PTH. The relationship between plasma Ca^{2+} concentration and PTH secretion by the parathyroid gland is shown in Fig. 6-10. In the normal range of plasma ionized Ca^{2+}, the secretion of PTH is inversely related to the plasma Ca^{2+} concentration; that is, decreased plasma Ca^{2+} concentration increases the secretion of PTH. Conversely, increased plasma Ca^{2+} suppresses the release of PTH. Thus, alterations in plasma Ca^{2+} result in primary changes in PTH secretion by the parathyroid gland. PTH acts directly on the bone and the kidney and indirectly on the GI tract to bring plasma Ca^{2+} concentration back to normal. Also shown in Fig. 6-10 is the relationship between plasma Ca^{2+} concentration and calcitonin (sometimes called thyrocalcitonin): secretion of calcitonin increases when plasma Ca^{2+} increases. When first identified, it was thought that calcitonin acted in concert with PTH to regulate plasma Ca^{2+} concentration. However, subsequent research has shown that while calcitonin may be important in other species, it is relatively unimportant in the regulation of plasma Ca^{2+} concentration in humans; therefore, calcitonin is ignored in the rest of this discussion.

FIGURE 6-10 ▶
Relationship between Plasma Ca^{2+} and Secretion of Parathyroid Hormone (PTH) and Calcitonin. *Secretion of PTH by the parathyroid gland is inversely related to plasma Ca^{2+} concentration.*

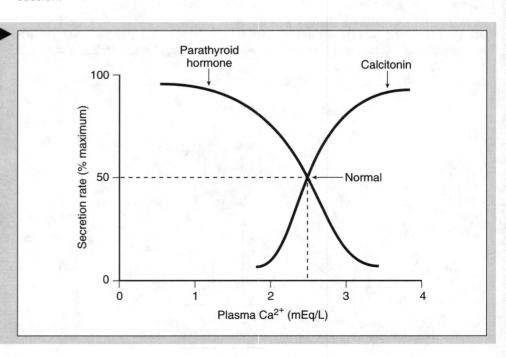

ACTIONS OF PARATHYROID HORMONE

Bone

The effect of PTH on bone is to increase the resorption of $CaHPO_4$. Thus resorption of bone results in an increased plasma concentration of Ca^{2+} and HPO_4^{2-}. In the plasma there is an equilibrium between $H_2PO_4^-$ and HPO_4^{2-}, depending on the existing H^+ concentration. Although at a normal plasma H^+ concentration over 80% of the PO_4 exists as HPO_4^{2-} rather than $H_2PO_4^-$, most clinical laboratories report phosphate concentration in the plasma as total phosphorus to avoid the confounding issue of the plasma H^+ concentration.

Contrary to popular thought, bone is not static but undergoes constant turnover. There is continuous resorption and deposition, and as much as 15% of the bone may turnover in 1 year. The repair of a fracture is a good example of deposition. As shown in Fig. 6-11, there are two active processes in equilibrium that determine bone turnover rate. Osteoblasts promote bone deposition, while osteoclasts continually promote bone resorption. Osteoblasts lay down a $CaHPO_4$ complex on the surface of the bone and migrate into the bone to form osteocytes. The $CaHPO_4$ complex in bone exists in two states. Before the bone matrix is fully established, the $CaHPO_4$ is in soluble form. As the bone matrix is being formed, the $CaHPO_4$ complex is incorporated into a cellular matrix that consists mostly of collagen. Osteoclasts are polynuclear cells that secrete acids and hydrolytic enzymes, which dissolve the matrix and release the bone mineral into the ECF. The osteoblasts continually repair the bone loss resulting from the osteoclasts.

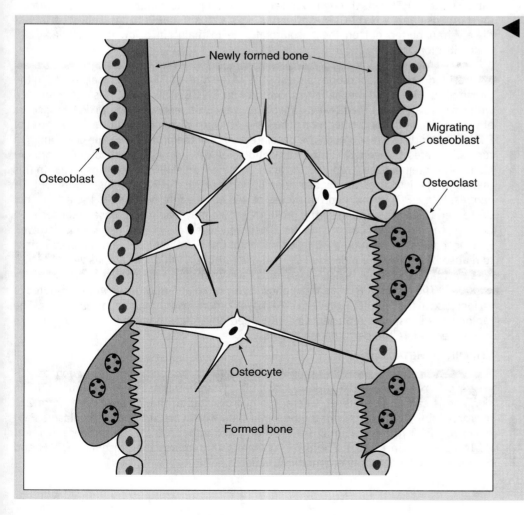

FIGURE 6-11
Factors Responsible for Bone Turnover.
Osteoblasts lay down the mineral and matrix in bone; osteoclasts dissolve the mineral and matrix in bone. Under normal conditions there is equilibrium between the two processes.

PTH has two actions on the bone. The first is to increase the resorption of the soluble form of $CaHPO_4$. The second function is to increase the action of the osteoclasts and increase the resorption of the bone matrix. The resorption of the soluble form of $CaHPO_4$ requires only minutes to hours, while the activation of osteoclasts requires hours to days. The net effect is to increase the concentration of both Ca^{2+} and HPO_4^{2-} in the plasma. Thus, a decrease in plasma Ca^{2+}, which results in an increase in PTH secretion by the parathyroid gland, leads to an increase in resorption of Ca^{2+} and HPO_4^{2-} from the bone. The increased plasma concentration of Ca^{2+} and HPO_4^{2-} results in an increase in the filtered load of both ions in the kidney. PTH affects the renal transport of both Ca^{2+} and HPO_4^{2-} and, therefore, adjusts the final plasma concentrations of both ions.

PTH increases the resorption of Ca^{2+} and HPO_4^{2-} from bone.

Kidney

CALCIUM AND PHOSPHATE TRANSPORT

PTH has two actions on the kidney. The first is to alter transport by increasing the reabsorption of Ca^{2+} and decreasing the reabsorption of HPO_4^{2-}. Calcium is reabsorbed along the entire length of the nephron. However, the site of hormonal regulation is the distal nephron. As Na^+ and water reabsorption occurs along the length of the proximal tubule, the concentration of Ca^{2+} in the tubular fluid increases, and Ca^{2+} is passively reabsorbed. Therefore, changes in Na^+ and water reabsorption in the proximal tubule may alter Ca^{2+} reabsorption through their effects on luminal Ca^{2+} concentration. In the thick ascending limb of the loop of Henle, Ca^{2+} is reabsorbed paracellularly down the electrochemical gradient resulting from the positive charge in the tubular lumen. As shown in Fig. 6-12A, PTH has a direct effect to increase Ca^{2+} reabsorption in the distal tubule system. PTH acts through cyclic adenosine monophosphate (cAMP) to stimulate a Ca^{2+}-ATPase and a Na^+–Ca^{2+}-antiporter. As Ca^{2+} diffuses into the cell, it is immediately transported out on the basolateral side to maintain a low intracellular Ca^{2+} concentration.

PTH increases the reabsorption of Ca^{2+} by the distal nephron segments.

PTH also acts on the kidney to decrease HPO_4^{2-} reabsorption by the proximal tubule. Under normal conditions almost 90% of the filtered HPO_4^{2-} is reabsorbed in the proximal tubule by the mechanism shown in Fig. 6-12B. The HPO_4^{2-} is cotransported with Na^+ via an apical membrane transporter. Very little reabsorption of HPO_4^{2-} occurs along the remainder of the nephron. The Na^+–HPO_4^{2-}-symporter is under the control of PTH. PTH binds to a receptor on the basolateral side of the proximal tubule cell, which in turn stimulates the generation of intracellular cAMP, leading to activation of protein kinase A. Protein kinase A reduces the activity of the Na^+–HPO_4^{2-}-cotransporter. In this manner, PTH decreases the reabsorption of both Na^+ and HPO_4^{2-}. High levels of PTH can result in HPO_4^{2-} excretion in excess of 40% of the filtered load. To the extent that decreased Na^+ reabsorption by the proximal tubule may lead to decreased reabsorption of Ca^{2+}, the delivery of Ca^{2+} to the distal nephron segments may be increased. However, in almost all cases the increased reabsorption of Ca^{2+} in the distal nephron is sufficient to reabsorb not only the increased Ca^{2+} delivered but additional Ca^{2+} as well. The net result is that PTH results in decreased renal Ca^{2+} excretion and increased renal HPO_4^{2-} excretion. The effect of PTH on the kidney is very rapid and may occur within minutes of an increase in the circulating levels of PTH, well before resorption of bone can occur. The rapidity of the response represents a classic feedforward mechanism in which a response is initiated before the perturbation occurs.

PTH decreases the cotransport of Na^+ and HPO_4^{2-} in the proximal tubule.

VITAMIN D METABOLISM

The second major action of PTH in the kidney is to promote the conversion of 25-hydroxyvitamin D_3 to 1,25-dihydroxyvitamin D_3. Vitamin D is activated by sunlight in the skin and is carried to the liver, where it is hydroxylated at the 25 position to form 25-hydroxyvitamin D_3. Enzymes in the proximal tubule cells are stimulated by plasma PTH to convert 25-hydroxyvitamin D_3 to 1,25-dihydroxyvitamin D_3. Thus the conversion of 25-hydroxyvitamin D_3 to 1,25-dihydroxyvitamin D_3 requires the presence of PTH and functional proximal tubule enzymatic function.

PTH stimulates the enzymatic rate of conversion of 25-hydroxyvitamin D_3 to 1,25-dihydroxyvitamin D_3 in the kidney.

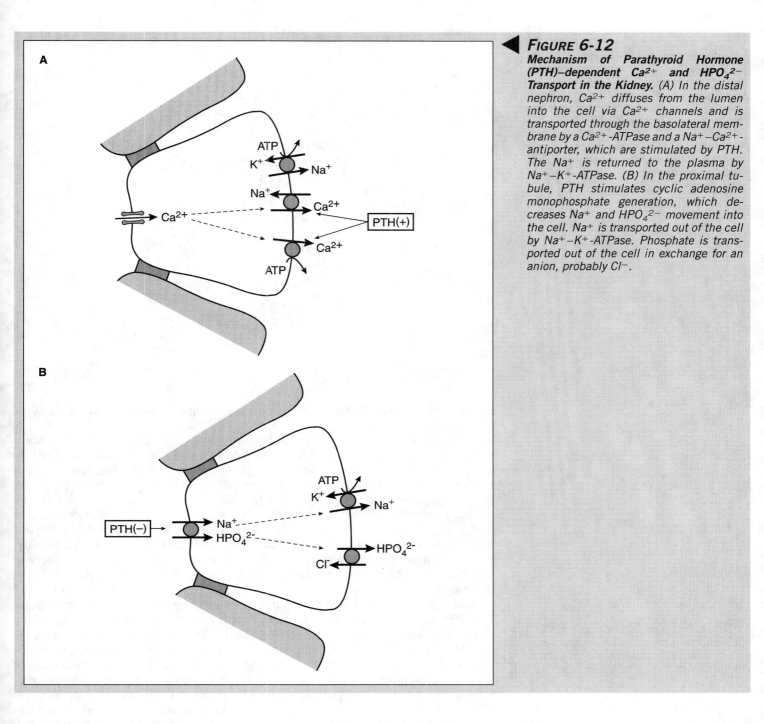

FIGURE 6-12
Mechanism of Parathyroid Hormone (PTH)–dependent Ca^{2+} and HPO_4^{2-} Transport in the Kidney. (A) In the distal nephron, Ca^{2+} diffuses from the lumen into the cell via Ca^{2+} channels and is transported through the basolateral membrane by a Ca^{2+}-ATPase and a $Na^+ - Ca^{2+}$-antiporter, which are stimulated by PTH. The Na^+ is returned to the plasma by $Na^+ - K^+$-ATPase. (B) In the proximal tubule, PTH stimulates cyclic adenosine monophosphate generation, which decreases Na^+ and HPO_4^{2-} movement into the cell. Na^+ is transported out of the cell by $Na^+ - K^+$-ATPase. Phosphate is transported out of the cell in exchange for an anion, probably Cl^-.

Gastrointestinal Tract

While the kidney regulates total body Na^+ and K^+ by adjusting the excretion to match the intake, changes in Ca^{2+} intake do not necessarily lead to changes in total body Ca^{2+}. The rate of Ca^{2+} absorption by the intestine is regulated by the plasma concentration of 1,25-dihydroxyvitamin D_3. Although the precise mechanism of Ca^{2+} absorption by the intestine is still being debated, the most likely mechanism is shown in Fig. 6-13. Ca^{2+} binds with an intestinal membrane Ca^{2+}-binding protein (IMCaBP) located on the luminal membrane of the intestinal cell. Because the intracellular Ca^{2+} concentration is very low relative to the luminal fluid concentration, the IMCaBP facilitates the diffusion of Ca^{2+} down its concentration gradient and into the cell. Once inside the cell, the Ca^{2+} is immediately sequestered by a Ca^{2+}-binding protein (CaBP). To prevent untoward increases in free intracellular Ca^{2+} concentration, the Ca^{2+} that is bound to CaBP, is

Intestinal absorption of Ca^{2+} is stimulated by 1,25-dihydroxyvitamin D_3.

FIGURE 6-13 ▶

Mechanism of Ca²⁺ Absorption by the Intestine. *The Ca²⁺ binds with intestinal membrane Ca²⁺-binding protein (IMCaBP) and diffuses into the cell, where it is bound and moved through the cell by Ca²⁺-binding protein (CaBP). Calcium is transported out of the cell by Ca²⁺-ATPase. All three components of this transport system are enhanced (+) by 1,25-dihydroxyvitamin D_3 (1,25-[OH]₂ D_3).*

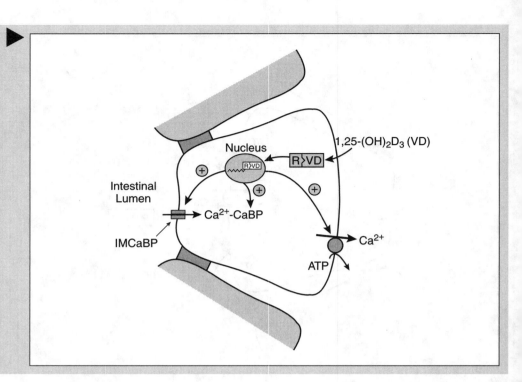

PTH indirectly controls the rate of Ca²⁺ absorption in the intestine by controlling the rate of production of 1,25-dihydroxyvitamin D_3 by the kidney.

moved through the cell cytosol to the basolateral membrane and transported out of the cell by a Ca²⁺-ATPase.

Also shown in Fig. 6-13, 1,25-dihydroxyvitamin D_3 regulates intestinal Ca²⁺ transport at three sites. It stimulates the production of both IMCaBP and CaBP to promote movement of Ca²⁺ into and through the cell. It also increases the activity of the Ca²⁺-ATPase to transport Ca²⁺ out of the cell. All three factors increase the rate of Ca²⁺ absorption by the intestine. The receptors for 1,25-dihydroxyvitamin D_3 are located inside the cells. Since 1,25-dihydroxyvitamin D_3 is a steroid hormone, it is free to diffuse into the cell. Receptor stimulation results in the production of RNA and subsequent synthesis of protein. Similar to most steroid hormones, 1,25-dihydroxyvitamin D_3 may require several hours to elicit the maximal response, and the response may last several hours after the plasma concentration of 1,25-dihydroxyvitamin D_3 has decreased.

It might be logical to assume that if PTH regulates renal function and bone resorption, PTH should also affect the GI tract. That is only partially true. PTH may have a marked effect on intestinal Ca²⁺ absorption, but the effect is *indirect*. If renal function is normal, plasma PTH is the rate-limiting step in the renal conversion of 25-hydroxyvitamin D_3 to 1,25-dihydroxyvitamin D_3. By controlling the rate of production of 1,25-dihydroxyvitamin D_3 in the kidney, PTH indirectly controls the rate of Ca²⁺ absorption by the intestine. Many years ago, before the effect of 1,25-dihydroxyvitamin on the GI tract was understood, a common problem in patients with severe renal disease was bone fractures. Sufficient plasma PTH was available, but the loss of renal mass resulted in a deficit in the production of functional 1,25-dihydroxyvitamin D_3. In the absence of 1,25-dihydroxyvitamin D_3, the body was simply unable to absorb ingested Ca²⁺. Even in severe renal failure there is still some urinary loss of Ca²⁺ by the kidney. In the absence of a GI input, the only source of plasma Ca²⁺ to replace the loss became the bone. There are currently a host of vitamin D derivatives available for treatment.

INTEGRATED RESPONSE TO HYPOCALCEMIA

As mentioned in the beginning of this section, the regulation of plasma Ca^{2+} concentration requires the integrated action of many systems in the body. Perhaps these actions can be best appreciated by using an example of the response to an acute decrease in plasma Ca^{2+} (Fig. 6-14). A decrease in plasma Ca^2 concentration results in an increase in PTH secretion from the parathyroid glands. The immediate effect of the increased plasma PTH is on the kidney to increase Ca^{2+} reabsorption by the distal nephrons and to decrease both Na^+ and $HPO_4{}^{2-}$ reabsorption by the proximal tubule. Simultaneously, PTH stimulates the release of soluble $CaHPO_4$ from the bone and thus tends to increase the concentrations of both Ca^{2+} and $HPO_4{}^{2-}$ in the plasma. PTH also stimulates the osteoclasts to result in sustained resorption of $CaHPO_4$ from the bone matrix. The utility of increasing the reabsorption of filtered Ca^{2+} is obvious. In the presence of an increased plasma Ca^{2+} concentration and, therefore, increased filtered load of Ca^{2+}, the reabsorption of Ca^{2+} must be increased to prevent the loss of Ca^{2+} in the urine. However, the advantage of decreasing the reabsorption of filtered $HPO_4{}^{2-}$ is not so obvious. In fact, the normal plasma concentrations of Ca^{2+} and $HPO_4{}^{2-}$ are close to saturation. This means that an increase in the concentration of both could lead to precipitation of a $CaHPO_4$ complex. (This chemical property actually facilitates the deposition of $CaHPO_4$ as hydroxyapatite in bone.) However, this also presents a potential problem to the body. If the concentrations of Ca^{2+} and $HPO_4{}^{2-}$ in the plasma markedly increase, the possibility of untoward $CaHPO_4$ precipitation in the plasma increases. The rapid effect of PTH on the kidney to increase $HPO_4{}^{2-}$ excretion will not only prevent a rise in plasma $HPO_4{}^{2-}$ but actually result in a *decrease* in plasma $HPO_4{}^{2-}$ concentration. Thus the renal response to a hypocalcemia-induced increase in plasma PTH results in a return of plasma Ca^{2+} concentration to normal and an acute decrease in plasma $HPO_4{}^{2-}$ concentration.

In addition to altering renal transport, PTH stimulates the enzymatic conversion of 25-hydroxyvitamin D_3 to 1,25-dihydroxyvitamin D_3. In the long term, the stimulation of Ca^{2+} absorption by 1,25-dihydroxyvitamin D_3 returns the total body stores of Ca^{2+} to normal. Thus, the plasma Ca^{2+} concentration is returned to normal, and the Ca^{2+} resorbed from the bone can be replaced.

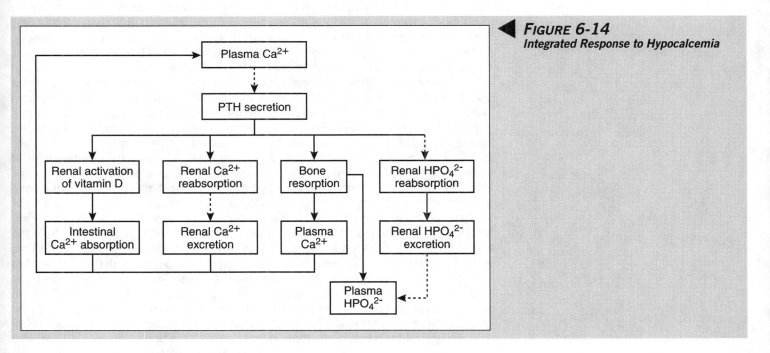

◀ *FIGURE 6-14*
Integrated Response to Hypocalcemia

RESOLUTION OF CLINICAL CASES

Case 1

The 55-year-old woman was exhibiting many of the symptoms of uncontrolled diabetes mellitus. Presumably as a result of the severe cold, she was unable to maintain the dietary regime and oral hypoglycemic treatment that was necessary to control the diabetes. The primary indicator of uncontrolled diabetes was the extremely high plasma glucose concentration and the high glucose content of the urine. Glucose appears in the urine because the high plasma glucose leads to a high filtered load that simply overwhelms the tubular transport maximum for glucose. Plasma K^+ concentration is in the hyperkalemic range. The initial reaction would be to assume that total body K^+ content is elevated. In fact this is probably not the case, rather there has been a redistribution and probably a net loss of K^+. First, high plasma glucose concentration creates an osmotic driving force for efflux of water out of the intracellular compartment. As a result, intracellular K^+ concentration rises, which in turn increases the efflux of K^+ into the ECF. Although probably not as important a factor in this particular case, the lack of insulin or reduced responsiveness to endogenous insulin also reduces the uptake of K^+ into intracellular stores.

Note that urine volume was also very high. The 1-hour collection of 250 mL translated to a daily urine output of 6 L, at least twice the normal value. This increased urine output was caused by the high filtered load of glucose, which acts as an osmotic diuretic, and the increased urine flow contributed to the high rate of K^+ excretion of 180 mEq/d. Mechanistically, this increased rate of excretion was due to elevated secretion into the cortical collecting tubule, which in turn was triggered by the high tubular fluid flow rate. Since this woman was not eating as a result of her cold, this rate of K^+ excretion almost certainly exceeded intake. Therefore, despite an elevated ECF K^+ concentration, her total body K^+ was probably reduced.

Case 2

The routine plasma analysis of the 45-year-old man was unremarkable. The plasma creatinine concentration was slightly elevated and the plasma HCO_3^- concentration was slightly decreased, but neither was clinically threatening. However, the plasma ionized Ca^{2+} was increased relative to normal (2.25–2.60 mEq/L), and the total phosphorus was concomitantly decreased relative to normal (2.7–4.5 mg/dl). An obvious dysfunction of the Ca^{2+}-regulating system was suspected. There were three possibilities. First, there could have been increased intestinal absorption of Ca^{2+}. However, if the PTH-renal axis was intact, the plasma PTH should have been decreased, and renal reabsorption of Ca^{2+} should have been minimal. Both actions should maintain the plasma Ca^{2+} around normal values. The second possibility was an inability of the kidney to excrete Ca^{2+} due to a decreased glomerular filtration rate. However, overall renal function was, at worst, only marginally compromised because the plasma concentrations of creatinine and BUN were near normal. The final possibility was the most likely cause of all the abnormalities. An elevated plasma PTH would have increased the rate of conversion of 25-hydroxyvitamin D_3 to 1,25-dihydroxyvitamin D_3 and led to increased intestinal absorption of Ca^{2+}. Excess PTH also would have increased resorption of $CaHPO_4$ from the bone and increased Ca^{2+} reabsorption by the kidney. All three effects would lead to the increased plasma Ca^{2+} concentration. Absorption of Ca^{2+} occurs in all parts of the bone including the joints, which explained the joint pain. Also, increased plasma Ca^{2+} decreased membrane excitability, and the difficulty in generating action potentials at the neuromuscular junction was responsible for the muscular weakness. That left the cause of the back pain to be elucidated. As discussed above, PTH leads to a decrease in Na^+ and HPO_4^{2-} reabsorption by the proximal tubule, which in turn increases Ca^{2+} delivery to the distal nephron. Under normal conditions, the increased Ca^{2+} reabsorption in the distal nephron is sufficient to compensate for the increased delivery and results in the net reabsorption of Ca^{2+} by the kidney. In this case, the filtered load was markedly increased because of the elevated plasma Ca^{2+} concentration. As a result of the high filtered load and depressed proximal reabsorption, the amount of Ca^{2+} delivered to the distal nephrons was so great that some of the filtered Ca^{2+} was not reabsorbed, and the Ca^{2+} in the urine increased along with the HPO_4^{2-}. One of the diagnostic features of hyperparathyroidism is hypercalciuria. If the increased concentrations of Ca^{2+} and HPO_4^{2-} are sufficiently high in the urine then $CaHPO_4$ precipitates and results in stone formation. The ureters are richly innervated with pain fibers, and kidney stones are very painful. Similar to most visceral pain, the pain from kidney stones is felt as diffuse pain, and the source of the pain is difficult to identify. Hence, the pain was described as lower back and scrotal. Small stones usually pass spontaneously into the urine without further complication. The patient was diagnosed as having an elevated PTH localized to a tumor of one of the parathyroid glands. The tumor was removed, and the symptoms resolved.

REVIEW QUESTIONS

1. In a patient with hyperkalemia, increased renal excretion of K^+ results primarily from
   - **(A)** increased filtered load of K^+
   - **(B)** decreased proximal tubule reabsorption of filtered K^+
   - **(C)** increased secretion of K^+ in the late distal and cortical collecting tubules
   - **(D)** decreased medullary collecting tubule K^+ reabsorption

2. Which combination of factors results in the greatest reduction in K^+ excretion?
   - **(A)** Low angiotensin II and metabolic acidosis caused by an inorganic acid
   - **(B)** Low angiotensin II and metabolic acidosis caused by an organic acid
   - **(C)** High angiotensin II and metabolic acidosis caused by an inorganic acid
   - **(D)** High angiotensin II and metabolic alkalosis

3. Which one of the following factors should reduce K^+ excretion?
   - **(A)** Loop diuretics
   - **(B)** Amiloride
   - **(C)** Metabolic alkalosis
   - **(D)** Increased plasma K^+

4. Which of the following *indirectly* results from increased plasma parathyroid hormone (PTH) concentration?
   - **(A)** Increased Ca^{2+} reabsorption by the distal nephron
   - **(B)** Decreased HPO_4^{2-} reabsorption by the proximal tubule
   - **(C)** Increased absorption of Ca^{2+} and HPO_4^{2-} from the bone
   - **(D)** Increased Ca^{2+} absorption by the intestines

5. Which of the following conditions would most likely lead to an increase in parathyroid hormone (PTH) secretion?
   - **(A)** Increased circulating concentration of 1,25-dihydroxyvitamin D_3
   - **(B)** Increased Ca^{2+} reabsorption by the kidney
   - **(C)** Decreased HPO_4^{2-} reabsorption by the kidney
   - **(D)** Decreased plasma Ca^{2+} concentration

6. Which is the most important regulator of plasma Ca^{2+} concentration?
   - **(A)** Parathyroid gland
   - **(B)** Kidney
   - **(C)** Gastrointestinal tract
   - **(D)** Bone

7. An injection of synthetic parathyroid hormone (PTH) would

   (A) increase plasma Ca^{2+} concentration and increase plasma HPO_4^{2-} concentration

   (B) increase plasma Ca^{2+} concentration and decrease plasma HPO_4^{2-} concentration

   (C) decrease plasma Ca^{2+} concentration and increase plasma HPO_4^{2-} concentration

   (D) decrease plasma Ca^{2+} concentration and decrease plasma HPO_4^{2-} concentration

8. The regulation of Ca^{2+} is unique compared to Na^+ and K^+ because

   (A) Ca^{2+} is regulated by hormones

   (B) both input and output are controlled

   (C) plasma concentration is unimportant

   (D) Ca^{2+} is dependent on dietary input

ANSWERS AND EXPLANATIONS

1. **The answer is C.** The late distal and cortical collecting tubules can adjust the rate of K^+ secretion over a wide range according to homeostatic demands. Given that 90% of the filtered load of K^+ is reabsorbed in segments prior to the distal nephron, yet an amount equal to 20% of the filtered load is excreted in the urine, even under normal circumstances, an amount of K^+ equivalent to 10% of the filtered load must have been secreted by the collecting tubule. Under hyperkalemic conditions, this value can increase to the point where the amount of K^+ excreted exceeds the amount filtered. Since the plasma concentration of K^+ has increased in this patient, the filtered load (GFR $\times$ P_K^+) has certainly increased (A). However, the contribution of an increased filtered load to the increased excretion is relatively small. Option B is probably incorrect. The amount of K^+ reabsorbed in the proximal tubule does not appear to change appreciably in response to changes in plasma K^+ status. Option D is probably also technically correct; however, the absolute rate of K^+ reabsorption in the collecting tubule is so low that any reduction in this process has relatively little effect on the amount of K^+ excreted.

2. **The answer is A.** The key to this question is to identify the combination of factors that reduces the electrochemical gradient that normally promotes K^+ secretion by the cortical collecting tubule. High angiotensin II leads to increased levels of aldosterone. This in turn stimulates Na^+–K^+-ATPase activity, which increases intracellular K^+ concentration and thus K^+ secretion. Hence, options C and D are incorrect. Options A and B both have low angiotensin levels, which is appropriate, but metabolic acidosis is caused by different types of acid. Recall that the rise in H^+ caused by an inorganic acid causes a greater cellular efflux of K^+ than a rise caused by an organic acid. The greater the efflux of K^+, the greater the reduction in intracellular K^+ concentration, which, at the level of the collecting tubule, would thereby oppose K^+ secretion. Therefore, option A is correct, since both factors reduce secretion and therefore excretion.

3. **The answer is B.** Amiloride blocks Na^+ channels on the luminal membrane of cortical collecting tubule cells. The consequent reduction in Na^+ reabsorption reduces the electrochemical driving force for K^+ secretion. First, the retention of Na^+ reduces the lumen-negative potential. Second, the reduced cellular uptake of Na^+ across the luminal membrane suppresses Na^+–K^+-ATPase activity, which is regulated by intracellular Na^+ concentration. For options A, C, and D, K^+ excretion certainly increases.

With the loop diuretic, the increased distal tubule fluid flow rate increases K^+ secretion. In addition, there is a reduction in normal K^+ reabsorption by the thick ascending limb. With metabolic alkalosis, there is an enhanced cellular uptake of K^+, which, at the level of the cortical collecting tubule, leads to increased secretion. Finally, an increased plasma K^+ concentration also leads to increased cellular uptake of K^+ and thereby secretion as a result of stimulation of the Na^+–K^+-AtPase.

4. **The answer is D.** PTH indirectly increases the absorption of Ca^{2+} by increasing the rate of conversion of 25-hydroxyvitamin D_3 to 1,25-dihydroxyvitamin D_3 in the kidney. The 1,25-dihydroxyvitamin D_3 increases Ca^{2+} absorption by the intestines. The other choices are direct effects of PTH on the target organ.

5. **The answer is D.** Decreased plasma Ca^{2+} stimulates the release of PTH from the parathyroid gland. The other three choices are actions of PTH, not regulators of PTH secretion.

6. **The answer is A.** Parathyroid hormone (PTH) is the most important regulator of plasma Ca^{2+} concentration, and PTH comes from the parathyroid gland. All the others are important, but they are regulated directly or indirectly by PTH.

7. **The answer is B.** PTH stimulates the kidney to increase Ca^{2+} reabsorption and decrease HPO_4^{2-} reabsorption. The initial stimulus to the bone is to increase the absorption of both Ca^{2+} and HPO_4^{2-}, which tends to raise the plasma concentration of both. However, the increased Ca^{2+} reabsorption in the kidney sustains the increase in plasma Ca^{2+} concentration while decreased HPO_4^{2-} reabsorption in the kidney leads to increased HPO_4^{2-} excretion and a decrease in plasma HPO_4^{2-} concentration.

8. **The answer is B.** Input of Ca^{2+} to the body is controlled by the effect of 1,25-dihydroxyvitamin D_3 on the intestine, and output is controlled by the effect of PTH on the kidney. Both Na^+ and K^+ are also influenced by the hormone aldosterone. Plasma concentrations of all three electrolytes are very important in physiologic function. The physiologic control systems that regulate Na^+ and K^+ respond to changes in dietary intake of Na^+ and K^+, while Ca^{2+} absorption in the intestine is generally independent of dietary intake.

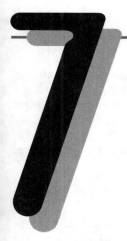

MAINTENANCE OF ACID–BASE BALANCE

CHAPTER OUTLINE

INTRODUCTION OF CLINICAL CASE

A known diabetic patient with a recent history of pneumonia was admitted to the emergency room. He was drowsy and confused. His respiratory rate was approximately 22 breaths/min, and he had a systolic blood pressure of 110 mm Hg with a diastolic of 65 mm Hg. A venous blood sample was drawn and sent for analysis. In the intervening hour he voided about 250 mL of urine. The venous blood sample gave the following data: sodium (Na^+), 130 mEq/L; potassium (K^+), 6.0 mEq/L; chloride (Cl^-), 98 mEq/L; bicarbonate (HCO_3^- [estimated]), 8 mEq/L; glucose, 800 mg/dL; creatinine, 1.2 mg/dL; and blood urea nitrogen (BUN), 18 mg/dL. A subsequent arterial blood sample gave the following additional data: oxygen partial pressure (Po_2), 95 mm Hg; carbon dioxide partial pressure (Pco_2), 20 mm Hg; hydrogen ion concentration (pH/H^+), 7.10/68.6 nmol/L; and HCO_3^- (calculated), 7 mEq/L.

ACID–BASE BALANCE

Source of the Hydrogen Ion

> *Free H^+ concentration in plasma is very low. It averages about 40 nmol/L compared to a plasma Na^+ concentration of 140,000,000 nmol/L.*

Similar to most electrolytes, H^+ concentration in the body is governed by a balance between intake and output. Although some free H^+ is ingested in the food we eat, most H^+ in the body is generated indirectly in the cells from metabolism of the ingested nutrients. It is the *free* H^+ concentration (measured as pH in the body) that is physiologically important. H^+ contained in foodstuff or water is of no consequence. For example, water exists as H_2O, and the H^+ is not free but bound. However, metabolism in the cells generates free H^+. It should be noted here that the free plasma H^+

concentration is exceedingly small when compared to other electrolytes. At a normal plasma pH of 7.4, the free H^+ concentration is 0.000040 mmol/L compared, for instance, to the plasma Na^+ concentration of 140 mmol/L. In user friendly terms, this is 40 nmol/L compared to the same Na^+ concentration of 140,000,000 nmol/L.

Following a meal, carbohydrates, proteins, and fats are metabolized. The metabolism of carbohydrates (CH_2O) in the cells can potentially generate a large supply of free H^+, according to the relationship below.

$$CH_2O + O_2 \rightarrow H_2O + CO_2 \underset{CA}{\overset{CA}{\rightleftharpoons}} H^+ + HCO_3^-$$

Oxygen (O_2) in the cell combines with the carbohydrate to form energy and leads to the generation of water (H_2O) and carbon dioxide (CO_2). The CO_2 and H_2O diffuse into the red blood cell (RBC) that supplied the O_2. In the presence of carbonic anhydrase (CA), the CO_2 and H_2O are reversibly converted to $H^+ + HCO_3^-$. The amount of free H^+ generated from the degradation of carbohydrates alone can generate as much as 20,000,000,000 nmol/d of H^+. Because of the continued necessary utilization of carbohydrates for energy, the above reaction is continuously forced to the right, and free H^+ is produced.

> *Metabolism of nutrients in the cells can produce as much as 20,000,000,000 nmol of free H^+ a day.*

Similar considerations may be applied to lipids and proteins, but many lipids and proteins also contain phosphate and sulfate, which are eventually metabolized to phosphoric and sulfuric acid (H_3PO_4 and H_2SO_4). Consider, for example, the complete degradation of the amino acid cysteine given below.

$$2 \, C_3H_7NO_2S + 12 \, O_2 \rightarrow CO(NH_2)_2 + 2 \, H^+ + 2 \, HSO_4^- + 5 \, CO_2 + 3 \, H_2O$$

Following deamination and conversion of the ammonia to urea, the remaining carbon moieties are metabolized normally. However, the inorganic residues remain as inorganic acids. In many Western societies, where meat is a major source of food intake, as many as 60,000,000 additional nmol/d of organic and inorganic acids may be produced from protein metabolism.

Since the extracellular fluid (ECF) contains only about 40 nmol/L of H^+, it is easy to appreciate that the total amount of H^+ contained in the extracellular fluid volume is very small compared to the amount of H^+ produced every day from ingested foods. Similarly, the maximum urine concentration of free H^+ is only 40,000 nmol/L. While this concentration is very large compared to the extracellular concentration, it is many orders of magnitude less than the potential free H^+ produced daily. The problem the body faces daily is twofold: (1) to minimize the increase in plasma H^+ generated from metabolism and (2) eventually, to eliminate it from the body. There are three major systems involved in the regulation of H^+ balance. The buffer systems of the body minimize the change in free H^+ concentration, the lungs eliminate the H^+ derived from CO_2, and the kidneys excrete the inorganic acids.

> *The buffer systems, the lungs, and the kidneys act in an integrated fashion to minimize any change in free H^+ concentration.*

Buffer Systems

MECHANISMS OF ACTION

In the simplest terms, a buffer is a molecule that combines with or releases a H^+. A classic illustration of this relationship is the dibasic-monobasic phosphate buffer system shown in the relationships below.

> *A buffer (Buf) system minimizes a change in free H^+ by accepting or donating a free H^+ according to the equilibrium relationship $H^+ + Buf^- \leftrightarrow HBuf$.*

$$H^+ + HPO_4^{2-} \longleftrightarrow H_2PO_4^- \tag{1}$$

$$\uparrow H^+ + HPO_4^{2-} \rightarrow H_2PO_4^- \tag{2}$$

$$\downarrow H^+ + HPO_4^{2-} \leftarrow H_2PO_4^- \tag{3}$$

As shown in relationship (1), at any given pH there is an equilibrium between the H^+, the dibasic phosphate (HPO_4^{2-}), and the monobasic phosphate ($H_2PO_4^-$). If H^+ is added, as shown in (2), the added H^+ combines with the HPO_4^{2-} to form $H_2PO_4^-$ and drives the relationship to the right. The increase in free H^+ is minimized. On the other hand, if H^+

is removed from the solution, as shown in (3), the $H_2PO_4^-$ dissociates and moves the reaction to the left. H^+ is added to minimize the decrease in free H^+. Thus whether H^+ is added to or removed from the solution, the buffer system minimizes the change in free H^+.

It must be emphasized that buffers cannot totally prevent a change in H^+ concentration. No buffer is 100% efficient, and therefore the H^+ concentration changes, but to a much smaller degree than if the buffer were not present. For example, assume that the HPO_4^{2-} in relationship (2) above has the ability to bind 98% of the added H^+. If 100 mmol of H^+ is added to 100 mmol of HPO_4^{2-}, the H^+ is buffered as shown below.

$$100\ H^+ + 100\ HPO_4^{2-} \rightarrow 2\ H^+ + 2\ HPO_4^{2-} + 98\ H_2PO_4^-$$

Most of the H^+ combines with the HPO_4^{2-} to form $H_2PO_4^-$. In the absence of the HPO_4^{2-}, the addition of 100 mmol of H^+ would have markedly increased the acidity of the solution by 100 mmol. However, in the presence of the HPO_4^{2-}, the added H^+ was buffered, the acidity increased by only 2 mmol or 2%, and the change in free H^+ was minimized. An added consequence of buffering is that the concentration of the HPO_4^{2-} decreased and the concentration of the $H_2PO_4^-$ increased. It should also be obvious that the capacity of the system to buffer is severely diminished. Addition of excess H^+ would greatly increase the free H^+ concentration because no HPO_4^{2-} would be available to bind the added H^+.

Although the ability to bind or release H^+ is dependent on the physical-chemical properties of the individual buffer system, the capacity to buffer is dependent on the relative concentration of the buffer pair. This relationship for the phosphate buffer system is illustrated in Fig. 7-1. In a solution with a very low H^+ concentration (high pH), almost all of the $H_2PO_4^-$ dissociates so that most phosphate exists as HPO_4^{2-} and very little as $H_2PO_4^-$. Thus the ratio of the concentrations of $H_2PO_4^-/HPO_4^{2-}$ is very low. At a pH of 10, the ratio is approximately 1/1500. If H^+ is added the pH will fall, but much of the H^+ will combine with the HPO_4^{2-} to form $H_2PO_4^-$. Although the change in free H^+ will be buffered, it will not be totally prevented, and the pH will fall. The pH at which the concentration of $H_2PO_4^-$ and HPO_4^{2-} are equal (concentration ratio = 1) is termed the pK. For the phosphate buffer system the pK is 6.8 and is the pH at which the capacity to buffer is greatest. As shown in Fig. 7-1, between a pH of 6 to 8 a large amount of HPO_4^{2-} can be converted to $H_2PO_4^-$, and the concentration ratio changes markedly before the pH changes to a significant degree. As more H^+ is added, conversion of HPO_4^{2-} to $H_2PO_4^-$ continues until the concentration of HPO_4^{2-} falls. In the example given, at a pH of 4 the concentration ratio of $H_2PO_4^-/HPO_4^{2-}$ is approximately 1500/1. At very low pH there is simply insufficient HPO_4^{2-} to accept any added H^+, and the capacity of the system to buffer falls significantly.

IMPORTANT BUFFERS

There are as many buffers in the body as there are compounds that can accept or donate free H^+. As individual buffer systems the physical-chemical characteristics differ, and the pK at which they operate most efficiently also varies. The combination of all buffers determines the free H^+ concentration. A partial listing of some important buffers is given in Table 7-1.

◀ **TABLE 7-1**
Important Buffers

Buffer	Mechanism	Site of Action
Phosphate	$H^+ + HPO_4^{2-} \leftrightarrow H_2PO_4^-$	Plasma and urine
Protein	$Prot^- + H^+ \leftrightarrow ProtH$	Intracellular
Organic phosphate	$H^+ + R{-}HPO_4^{2-} \leftrightarrow R{-}H_2PO_4^-$	Intracellular
Hemoglobin	$HbO_2 \rightarrow Hb^- + O_2 + H^+ \leftrightarrow HbH + O_2$	Red cells
Hydroxyapatite	$Ca_n(PO_4)_nO_2H^- + H^+ \leftrightarrow Ca_n(PO_4)_n(OH)_2$	Bone
Carbon dioxide–bicarbonate	$H_2O + CO_2 \overset{CA}{\rightleftharpoons} H^+ + HCO_3^-$	Extracellular

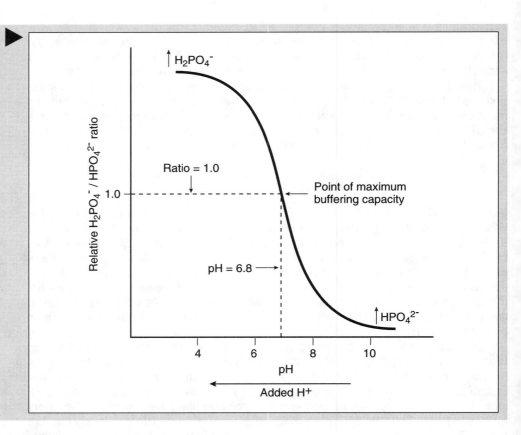

In addition to buffering in the plasma, the phosphate buffer system plays a major role in the excretion of bound H^+ in the urine. Both proteins and organic phosphates are major buffers in the cells. Hemoglobin has a major function to deliver O_2 to the cells for metabolism and to remove CO_2. However, deoxygenated hemoglobin has a marked affinity for H^+ when compared to oxygenated hemoglobin. It is the primary mechanism by which the H^+ generated from H_2O and CO_2 in the RBC is buffered. Hydroxyapatite is the primary component of bone and is mentioned only because of the large bone mass. Bone is not a particularly powerful buffer, but there is a lot of it in the body. As discussed below, the CO_2–HCO_3^- system is probably the most important of those listed.

CARBON DIOXIDE–BICARBONATE BUFFER SYSTEM

The CO_2–HCO_3^- buffer system is important for two reasons. The first is a matter of diagnosis in that all three components can be measured and quantitated. The second is of physiologic importance in that both CO_2 and HCO_3^- can be physiologically controlled. The CO_2 is determined by the lungs, while the plasma HCO_3^- is regulated by the kidneys.

Quantitation. In the presence of CA, there is a reversible reaction between $CO_2 + H_2O$ and $H^+ + HCO_3^-$.

$$H_2O + CO_2 \longleftrightarrow H^+ + HCO_3^-$$

Using the law of mass balance from elementary chemistry, a quantitative relationship between the reactants and the products can be written.

$$\frac{[H^+][HCO_3^-]}{[H_2O][CO_2]} = K$$

The concentration of H_2O is constant and can be ignored. If the relationship is rearranged to solve for H^+ and CO_2 is expressed as a partial pressure (P_{CO_2}), the result is the well-known Henderson equation.

$$H^+ = 24 \frac{P_{CO_2}}{HCO_3^-}$$

The CO_2–HCO_3^- buffer system is the most important buffer system in the body because it can be regulated. In the relationship $H_2O + CO_2 \leftrightarrow H^+ + HCO_3^-$, both the CO_2 and the HCO_3^- can be physiologically controlled.

If the arterial P_{CO_2} is expressed in mm Hg and the HCO_3^- in mEq/L, the constant (K) becomes 24, which directly returns the H^+ concentration in nmol/L. In normal conditions the P_{CO_2} is 40 mm Hg, the HCO_3^- concentration is 24 mEq/L, and the H^+ concentration is 40 nmol/L, which makes the constant 24 easy to remember. If any two are known, the other can be determined.

Since many clinical laboratories use pH instead of H^+ concentration, it is necessary to convert the Henderson equation from H^+ concentration to pH. It is a simple matter to take the $-\log$ of the Henderson equation and convert it to the Henderson-Hasselbalch equation. The $-\log$ of the H^+ concentration is the pH. The pH at which the concentration of CO_2 and HCO_3^- are equal is the pK, which for the case of the CO_2–HCO_3^- system is 6.1. Since the $-\log$ is taken, the ratio of CO_2 and HCO_3^- is reversed. Finally, because the log of the concentration ratios is taken, the arterial P_{CO_2} must be converted to CO_2 concentration. The solubility coefficient for CO_2 is 0.03 nmol/L per mm Hg of pressure. To obtain the concentration of CO_2, simply multiply the arterial P_{CO_2} by 0.03. In its final form the Henderson-Hasselbalch equation becomes

$$pH = 6.1 + \log \frac{HCO_3^-}{0.03 \times P_{CO_2}}$$

It is not at all necessary to be able to derive either equation, but it is comforting to know that they can be obtained from simple physical and chemical principles.

Before proceeding, there are several considerations that may be of help in the future. First, it is imperative to obtain an appreciation of the role the respiratory and renal systems play in the regulation of H^+ concentration. It is sometimes helpful to express the Henderson-Hasselbalch equation as

$$pH = 6.1 + \log \frac{kidneys}{lungs}$$

since the kidneys are responsible for the regulation of HCO_3^- and the lungs are responsible for the regulation of the arterial P_{CO_2}. Second, many of us are uncomfortable working with logarithms. At a normal pH of 7.4, the ratio of the $(HCO_3^-)/(0.03 \times P_{CO_2})$ is 20/1: $(24\ mEq/L)/(0.03 \times 40\ mm\ Hg)$. Any ratio greater than 20/1 results in a pH greater than normal, and any ratio less than 20/1 results in a pH less than normal. Last, under normal physiologic conditions the relationship between pH and H^+ concentration can be approximated. A deviation from the normal physiologic arterial pH of 7.4 by 0.1 units is equivalent to a deviation of approximately 10 nmol/L in the normal H^+ concentration of 40 nmol/L. Thus a pH of 7.3 is approximately the same as a H^+ concentration of 50 nmol/L, and a pH of 7.5 is approximately the same as a H^+ concentration of 30 nmol/L. Since pH is a log function, it is obvious that the further one ventures from 7.4, the less exact the conversion.

Respiratory System

The respiratory system has several obvious functions. It supplies O_2 inspired in the lungs to the blood in the cardiovascular system, which is then transported to the tissue cells for utilization. It also removes the CO_2 that has been generated in the cells and then carried to the lungs. What is not intuitive is the role of the respiratory system in the regulation of plasma H^+ concentration. As pointed out earlier in the discussion on food metabolism, there is an equilibrium between $CO_2 + H_2O$ and $H^+ + HCO_3^-$ such that any change in CO_2 can result in a corresponding change in H^+ concentration. Since the arterial P_{CO_2} is regulated by the lungs, changes in respiratory function also lead to changes in H^+ concentration.

The respiratory system can affect the free H^+ concentration by altering the CO_2 component of the relationship $H_2O + CO_2 \leftrightarrow H^+ + HCO_3^-$.

HYDROGEN BUFFERING

Hemoglobin carries O_2 in the RBC from the lungs to the tissue cells for metabolism. As shown in Fig. 7-2, the O_2 dissociates from the hemoglobin and diffuses down its concentration gradient into the cell, where it is metabolized into energy and CO_2. The CO_2 diffuses from the tissue cell into the RBC, where it combines with H_2O in the presence of CA to form H^+ and HCO_3^-. The H^+ then combines with the deoxygenated hemoglobin where it is buffered, and thus the change in free H^+ is minimized. The

HCO_3^- formed in the cell diffuses into the plasma, and to maintain electrical neutrality, a Cl^- diffuses into the RBC. After the RBC is carried to the lungs, the process is reversed. In the alveoli the high O_2 causes diffusion into the RBC, where it oxygenates the hemoglobin and displaces the H^+. The H^+ then recombines with HCO_3^- that diffuses into the RBC from the plasma to form CO_2 and H_2O. The high CO_2 concentration in the RBC causes diffusion of CO_2 into the alveoli, where it is expired into the air.

FIGURE 7-2 ▶

Mechanism of Hemoglobin Buffering of H^+ Generated in the Tissues from Metabolism. The H^+ from the tissues combines with the hemoglobin (Hb) in the red blood cell. The H^+-hemoglobin (HHb) is carried to the lungs. O_2 displaces the H^+ from the hemoglobin. The H^+ combines with HCO_3^- to form CO_2 and H_2O. The CO_2 is expired in the lungs, and the H^+ returns to H_2O.

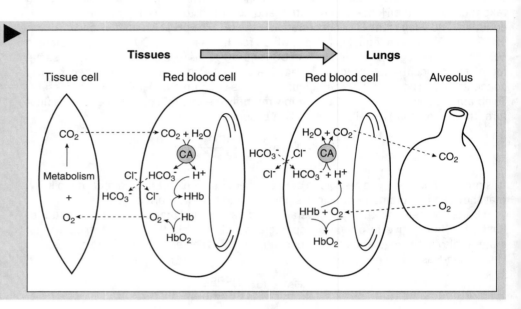

In the tissues, the reaction $H_2O + CO_2 \overset{CA}{\rightleftharpoons} H^+ + HCO_3^-$ is driven to the right because of continual generation of CO_2 and subsequent formation of H^+ and HCO_3^-. In the lungs, the reaction is driven to the left because of the removal of CO_2. In this manner the H^+ generated in the cells is buffered by hemoglobin, carried to the lungs, and excreted as CO_2 into the air. When it is considered that as much as 20,000,000,000 nmol of H^+ are generated from the metabolism of carbohydrates alone, a vast portion of the daily H^+ insult to the body is eliminated. It should be intuitively obvious that continual removal of CO_2 from the blood is necessary for normal H^+ metabolism. Indeed, an inability to expire CO_2, as occurs with many pulmonary diseases, may result in CO_2 retention and increased H^+ concentration. This condition is termed *respiratory acidosis*.

Hemoglobin has a unique characteristic that allows it to act as a very powerful buffer in the RBC. Deoxygenated hemoglobin has a much greater affinity for H^+ than oxygenated hemoglobin. This characteristic is illustrated in Fig. 7-3, which compares the buffering capacity of the two states at various degrees of acidity. When hemoglobin is deoxygenated, the relationship between pH and added H^+ shifts from oxygenated hemoglobin (A) to deoxygenated hemoglobin (B). Thus a large amount of H^+ can be added to the deoxygenated hemoglobin without a significant change in pH. This shift from oxygenated to deoxygenated hemoglobin, which occurs at the cellular level, allows H^+ to be buffered without significantly decreasing the pH of the venous blood. The amount of H^+ that can be buffered is dependent on the amount of hemoglobin in the blood. The decrease in hematocrit and hemoglobin that occurs in many patients with chronic renal failure may contribute to the acidosis seen in these patients.

> Deoxygenated hemoglobin has a greater affinity for H^+ than oxygenated hemoglobin. The H^+ generated in the tissues from metabolism is buffered by the deoxygenated hemoglobin and carried to the lungs.

CARBON DIOXIDE REGULATION

Since CO_2 is one-half of the CO_2–HCO_3^- buffer system, it is imperative that the body regulates the concentration of arterial CO_2. The body uses two major mechanisms to regulate the arterial Pco_2 (Fig. 7-4). An increase in arterial Pco_2 directly stimulates alveolar ventilation (Fig. 7-4A). In a classic negative feedback fashion, the increase in alveolar ventilation leads to an increase in CO_2 expiration and a subsequent return of arterial Pco_2 to normal (Fig. 7-4B). Increased H^+ also stimulates alveolar ventilation

(Fig. 7-4C). The increased alveolar ventilation decreases the arterial P_{CO_2}. The subsequent decrease in arterial P_{CO_2} also decreases the plasma H^+ concentration and represents the second negative feedback mechanism.

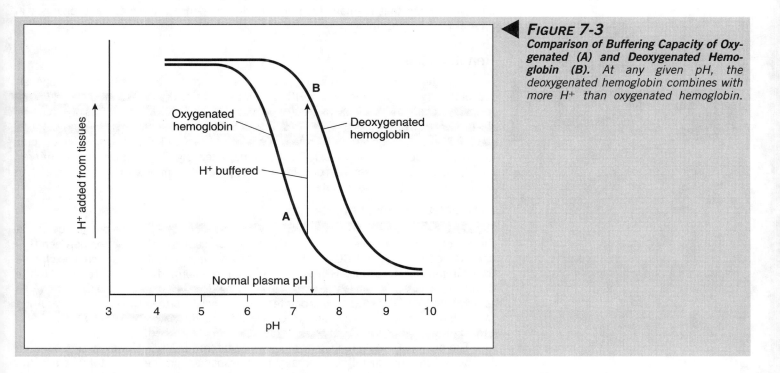

FIGURE 7-3
Comparison of Buffering Capacity of Oxygenated (A) and Deoxygenated Hemoglobin (B). At any given pH, the deoxygenated hemoglobin combines with more H^+ than oxygenated hemoglobin.

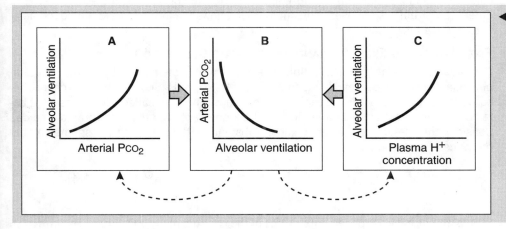

FIGURE 7-4
Relationship of the Major Mechanisms that Control Arterial P_{CO_2}. Increased P_{CO_2} stimulates alveolar ventilation (A). Increased H^+ also stimulates alveolar ventilation (C). At equilibrium, the two stimuli determine the alveolar ventilation (B). Alveolar ventilation ultimately determines the arterial P_{CO_2}, and the P_{CO_2} alters the plasma H^+ concentration.

There are conditions in which the two mechanisms work in concert and others when they are in conflict. It is easy to see that an increase in both arterial P_{CO_2} and H^+ concentration would lead to an additive effect since they both stimulate alveolar ventilation. However, there are times when the two act in opposite directions. Addition of H^+ to the plasma would lead to an increase in alveolar ventilation and a decrease in arterial P_{CO_2}. However, the decrease in arterial P_{CO_2} would tend to inhibit alveolar ventilation and prevent a further fall in arterial P_{CO_2} (see Fig. 7-4A). The final arterial P_{CO_2} is the result of the equilibrium reached between the two competing stimuli. Conversely, decreased H^+ tends to decrease alveolar ventilation and leads to an increase in P_{CO_2}. The increased P_{CO_2} stimulates alveolar ventilation and prevents a further increase in arterial P_{CO_2} until a new equilibrium is reached. A change in arterial H^+ concentration results in a change in respiratory function, which in turn alters the CO_2 component of the

Increased plasma H^+ concentration and increased arterial P_{CO_2} stimulate alveolar ventilation. Under normal conditions, the rate of alveolar ventilation controls the arterial P_{CO_2}.

CO_2–HCO_3^- buffer system. Inspection of the Henderson equation illustrates that changes in arterial P_{CO_2} can directly affect the H^+ concentration. An increased P_{CO_2} would result in increased H^+ concentration, while a decrease in arterial P_{CO_2} would result in decreased H^+ concentration. The body uses the interplay of the two physiologic control systems that regulate arterial P_{CO_2} to compensate for metabolic changes in arterial H^+ concentration.

Renal System

> *The kidney regulates plasma HCO_3^- concentration by secreting a H^+ ion into the tubular lumen and returning a HCO_3^- ion to the blood.*

HCO_3^- is the second half of the CO_2–HCO_3^- buffer system, and the kidney is responsible for the regulation of the plasma HCO_3^- concentration. The first role of the kidney is to reabsorb essentially all of the filtered HCO_3^- and prevent the untoward loss of HCO_3^- in the urine. The second and probably more important role of the kidney is to excrete H^+ in the urine and produce new HCO_3^-, which is returned to the blood. The excretion of acids and the production of new HCO_3^- occur simultaneously. The reabsorption of filtered HCO_3^- as well as the excretion of acids and the production of new HCO_3^- all depend on H^+ *secretion* by the renal tubule.

BICARBONATE REABSORPTION

To reabsorb a filtered HCO_3^-, the renal tubule must secrete a H^+. This process begins in the cell of the renal tubule (see Chap. 4). Cellular CA catalyzes the reaction between H_2O and CO_2 to form H^+ and HCO_3^-. The H^+ is secreted into the tubular lumen in exchange for a filtered Na^+ by a Na^+–H^+-exchanger. The newly formed HCO_3^- is returned to the blood. Once in the lumen, the H^+ combines with filtered HCO_3^- to form CO_2 and H_2O, which diffuse into the cell. As was pointed out, the newly formed HCO_3^- that is returned to the blood came from CO_2 and H_2O inside the cell, while the filtered HCO_3^- was converted to CO_2 and H_2O, which are subsequently reabsorbed.

The proximal tubule reabsorbs most of the filtered HCO_3^-. However, H^+ secretion still occurs in more distal nephron segments, especially in the distal tubules and the collecting tubule system. In the absence of HCO_3^- to combine with the secreted H^+, other tubular buffers are used. This interaction allows the kidney to excrete bound acid and produce new HCO_3^-.

FIXED HYDROGEN EXCRETION AND BICARBONATE GENERATION

Formation of Titratable Acids. Cellular metabolism of proteins and lipids that contain phosphate or sulfate can lead to the formation of H_3PO_4 or H_2SO_4. These acids cannot be converted to CO_2 and H_2O and expired by the lungs. These so-called fixed acids must be removed from the plasma by the kidney. The kidney excretes them as titratable acids. Consider the metabolism of an organic substance (R) containing phosphate in the presence of Na^+ and HCO_3^-:

$$R - H_2PO_4^- \rightarrow H^+ + HCO_3^- + Na^+ + HPO_4^{2-} \rightarrow CO_2 + H_2O + Na^+ + HPO_4^{2-}$$

Several things have happened. First, some of the H^+ from the $H_2PO_4^-$ has been buffered by the HCO_3^-, and the increase in free H^+ has been minimized. This example emphasizes the importance of HCO_3^- as a buffer. However, recall that buffering is not complete; it only minimizes the change in free H^+, and H^+ concentration does increase. Second, and perhaps almost as important, the HCO_3^- concentration has decreased. The HCO_3^- was consumed in the buffering process. To correct for the acid insult fully, the added H^+ must be excreted by the kidney and the consumed HCO_3^- must be replaced.

> *The kidney forms titratable acids by combining secreted H^+ with buffers in the tubular fluid. The titratable acids are then excreted in the urine.*

Metabolism of organic molecules containing fixed acids may contribute as much as 60 mmol/d of H^+ to the body, and it falls to the kidney to excrete many of them as titratable acids. In the example given above the opposite events occur in the kidney, which are summarized in Fig. 7-5. The general mechanism for the production of H^+ and HCO_3^- from CO_2 and H_2O exists in the distal nephron segments as well as in the proximal tubule. However, in the distal tubule and collecting system the tubular fluid HCO_3^- concentration is very low or zero because all the filtered HCO_3^- has been reabsorbed more proximally. The secreted H^+ now combines with a filtered HPO_4^{2-} to form $H_2PO_4^-$, which is excreted in the urine. The new HCO_3^- formed in the cell exits on the basolateral side and enters the blood to replace the HCO_3^-, which was used for buffering in other parts of the body. Because the renal cells continuously produce H^+, there is a continuous supply of H^+ to combine with the filtered HPO_4^{2-}. Since H^+ is secreted into the lumen of the tubule, the H^+ concentration in the tubular fluid increases and the pH falls, which favors the conversion of HPO_4^{2-} to $H_2PO_4^-$. In simple terms, the process may be thought of in two steps. The generation of fixed acids in the body are buffered and then carried to the kidney. The kidney then secretes H^+ that recombines with the acids, which are then excreted. In the process of secreting the H^+, the kidney simultaneously replenishes the plasma HCO_3^- used in the buffering. Although HPO_4^{2-} is the major titratable acid in the urine, any molecule that can combine with the secreted H^+, including creatinine, sulfate, and the anions of fatty acids, may serve the function of a titratable acid and be excreted in the urine.

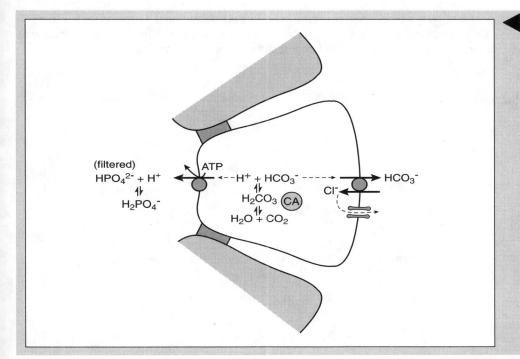

FIGURE 7-5
Mechanism of Formation of Titratable Acids in the Distal Nephron. The H^+ generated from CO_2 and H_2O by carbonic anhydrase (CA) in the cell is secreted into the tubule lumen via H^+-ATPase and combines with a titratable acid (HPO_4^{2-}). The HCO_3^- is returned to the blood. The net result is excretion of a bound H^+ and the formation of new HCO_3^-, which is added to the body.

(filtered)
$HPO_4^{2-} + H^+$
$\updownarrow$
$H_2PO_4^-$

ATP

$H^+ + HCO_3^-$
$\updownarrow$
H_2CO_3 (CA)
$\updownarrow$
$H_2O + CO_2$

Cl^-

HCO_3^-

Formation of Ammonium. It should be obvious that the amount of H^+ that can be excreted as titratable acid is limited by the amount of titratable acids filtered at the glomerulus and therefore available in the tubular fluid. Under normal conditions, the urine is very acidic compared to plasma and has a pH of about 5. Without something to accept the H^+, further H^+ secretion would bring the urine pH to an impossibly low level. A urine pH of 4.4 would present a 1000-fold H^+ gradient for diffusion into the plasma, which has a pH of 7.4. It is simply impossible for the cell to continue to secrete H^+ against such a large gradient. For continued secretion and excretion of H^+ to occur, an additional H^+ buffer must be present. The kidney has a somewhat unique mechanism by which it generates ammonia and uses it as a H^+ acceptor.

In the proximal tubule, the kidney generates ammonia (NH_3) from glutamine. The NH_3 generated is in equilibrium with ammonium ion (NH_4^+) and H^+ according to the reaction:

$$NH_3 + H^+ \longleftrightarrow NH_4^+$$

Because the pK of the reaction is about 9.2, most, but not all, of the buffer pair NH_3–NH_4^+ exists as NH_4^+. The NH_4^+ is secreted by the proximal tubule into the tubular fluid. However, the secreted NH_4^+ is subsequently reabsorbed by the medullary thick ascending

The kidney forms NH_4^+ in the tubule fluid by combining secreted H^+ with lipid soluble NH_3 generated by the renal tubule cells. The resulting NH_4^+ in the tubular fluid is lipid insoluble and is trapped. The NH_4^+ is then excreted in the urine.

Chronic increases in plasma H^+ stimulate the production of NH_3 by the renal tubule cells.

limb of the loop of Henle probably by substituting for Na^+ on the $Na^+-K^+-2Cl^-$-cotransporter. Then it is concentrated in the renal medullary interstitium (similar to Na^+).

In the medullary interstitium, the equilibrium between NH_4^+ and NH_3 still exists. At the collecting duct, the lipid soluble NH_3 diffuses from the interstitium into the lumen of the collecting duct, where it combines with a secreted H^+ generated from CO_2 and H_2O by the intercalated cells. This mechanism has been termed "diffusion trapping" (Fig. 7-6). The reason for the name is obvious. The NH_3 diffuses into the lumen and combines with the H^+ where it is trapped. Since the resulting NH_4^+ is lipid insoluble, it cannot diffuse back out of the tubule lumen. Because the NH_3 is continuously converted to NH_4^+, the resulting concentration gradient for NH_3 promotes continued diffusion of NH_3 from the interstitium into the tubular lumen. In addition to supplying an added buffer for secreted H^+ in normal conditions, the $NH_3-NH_4^+$ system serves as an important mechanism for increased H^+ secretion during times of chronic acid insult to the body. Prolonged acidosis stimulates the production of NH_4^+ by the proximal tubule. Since this is a biochemical process that probably requires enzyme induction, the full expression of increased NH_4^+ production may take hours to days. Although the process is slow to reach full development, it is a very important mechanism. Often NH_4^+ excretion increases severalfold during disease states that result in chronic systemic acidosis.

FIGURE 7-6
Mechanism of Formation of NH_4^+ in the Distal Nephron Segments. *The lipid soluble NH_3 diffuses from the interstitium through the cell membranes. The H^+ generated from CO_2 and H_2O by carbonic anhydrase (CA) in the cell is secreted into the tubule lumen. Because the H^+ concentration in the lumen is high, the H^+ combines with the NH_3 to form NH_4^+. The NH_4^+ is not soluble in the lipid cell membrane and is trapped in the lumen. The NH_4^+ is excreted, and the HCO_3^- is returned to the body as new HCO_3^-.*

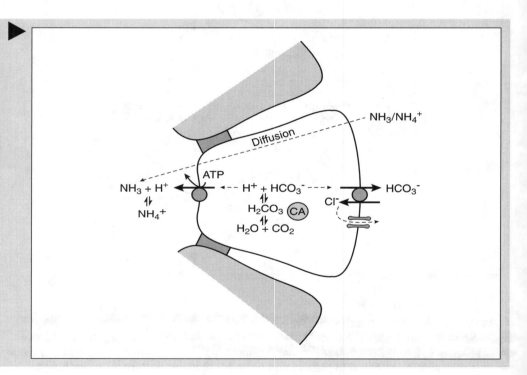

For every titratable acid and NH_4^+ excreted in the urine, a new HCO_3^- is added to the blood.

Two ideas are common to the mechanisms of H^+ secretion discussed above. First, the H^+ and HCO_3^- came from the combination of CO_2 and H_2O inside the cell. The H^+ was secreted, and the HCO_3^- was returned to the plasma. Any circumstance that accelerates the CO_2-H_2O reaction will increase the rate of both H^+ secretion and HCO_3^- generation. Second, and also important for the quantitation of renal H^+ handling, is that the secretion of one H^+ always results in the return of one HCO_3^- to the plasma. In the case of HCO_3^- conservation, the HCO_3^- from the cell replaces the filtered HCO_3^- that was consumed by the H^+ secreted into the lumen. In addition, it can be seen that for every titratable acid or NH_4^+ excreted in the urine, a H^+ had to be secreted into the tubular lumen. It is a simple matter to determine the rate of H^+ secretion by the determination of the rate of HCO_3^- reabsorption and the excretion rate of titratable acids and NH_4^+. It is also important to realize that the rate of excretion of titratable acid and

NH_4^+ is equivalent to the rate of new HCO_3^- generated by the kidney and returned to the body.

REGULATION OF HYDROGEN SECRETION

The regulation of plasma H^+ concentration in both health and disease depends on the integrated function of the buffer systems, the respiratory system, and the renal system. The ability of the buffer systems to minimize the change in free H^+ in the plasma is dependent on the amount of buffers in the body. The amount of each buffer, with the exception of CO_2–HCO_3^-, is usually fixed. While the buffer systems act rapidly, they have a finite capacity. The respiratory system also acts rapidly; respiratory adjustments can occur in a matter of minutes. However, the capacity of the respiratory system to adjust to acid–base changes is limited. The kidney is much slower to react but is much more powerful than the other two systems. Renal adjustments to acid–base changes depend on renal tubular secretion of H^+, and there are a large number of factors that alter the rate of H^+ secretion. The most important are:

1. Filtered HCO_3^-
2. Arterial Pco_2
3. Aldosterone
4. Proximal tubule Na^+ reabsorption
5. Plasma H^+ concentration

Filtered Bicarbonate. The primary function of the kidney in the regulation of acid–base balance is to conserve the body stores of HCO_3^- and maintain the plasma HCO_3^- concentration constant. Increases or decreases in plasma HCO_3^- result in changes in the amount of filtered HCO_3^-. For reasons discussed in earlier chapters, the kidney automatically adjusts the amount of HCO_3^- reabsorbed to match the amount filtered and maintains glomerulotubular balance (Fig. 7-7). It is easy to see how decreases in filtered HCO_3^- result in decreased HCO_3^- reabsorption. The H^+ secretion is sufficient to reabsorb all the filtered HCO_3^-. Although increased filtered HCO_3^- results in increased H^+ secretion and increased HCO_3^- reabsorption, this ability is limited. At very high plasma HCO_3^- concentrations the amount of HCO_3^- filtered exceeds the ability of the kidney to increase H^+ secretion, and some of the filtered HCO_3^- escapes reabsorption and is then lost in the urine. This inability to completely reabsorb all the filtered HCO_3^- explains why it is very difficult to increase plasma HCO_3^- concentration to high levels by the ingestion of HCO_3^- in the presence of a healthy kidney. Plasma HCO_3^- concentration does not usually increase appreciably, unless H^+ secretion is stimulated by other factors or the glomerular filtration rate (GFR) is simultaneously decreased.

> *Increased filtered HCO_3^- increases HCO_3^- reabsorption.*

Arterial Pco_2. Most of the H^+ secreted by the renal cells comes from the intracellular reaction $CO_2 + H_2O \leftrightarrow H^+ + HCO_3^-$. Since the reaction is in equilibrium, the production of H^+ available for secretion by the cells is increased by the addition of CO_2 to the system. The relationship between H^+ secretion and arterial Pco_2 is shown in Fig. 7-8. As the Pco_2 increases, the CO_2 concentration in the cell increases, and the above reaction is driven to the right to produce more H^+, which is subsequently secreted into the lumen. Conversely, a decrease in Pco_2 results in a decrease in H^+ secretion. The kidney's response to changes in Pco_2 is also an adaptive renal mechanism to respond to acid–base disturbances brought about by the lungs. An inability to expire CO_2, which might occur in obstructive lung disease, increases arterial Pco_2. The increased Pco_2 results in elevated systemic H^+ concentration. The increased Pco_2, which also stimulates the kidney to increase H^+ secretion and generate new HCO_3^- in response to the respiratory acidosis, is an important compensatory renal mechanism to minimize the change in free H^+ concentration. Similarly, hyperventilation lowers arterial Pco_2 and plasma H^+ concentration. The appropriate renal response to the decreased Pco_2 is to decrease H^+ secretion and generate less new HCO_3^- to minimize the change in free H^+ concentration.

> *Increased arterial Pco_2 increases renal tubular H^+ secretion and HCO_3^- generation.*

FIGURE 7-7 ▶

Relationship between Filtered HCO₃⁻ and H⁺ Secretion. *To maintain glomerulotubular balance, H⁺ secretion and HCO₃⁻ reabsorption decrease as the filtered load of HCO₃⁻ decreases. As filtered HCO₃⁻ increases above normal, glomerulotubular balance falls behind, and H⁺ secretion fails to keep up with all the filtered HCO₃⁻. In this case, some of the filtered HCO₃⁻ escapes reabsorption.*

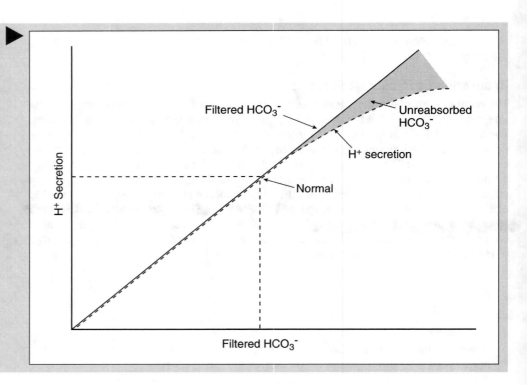

FIGURE 7-8 ▶

Relationship between Arterial Pco₂ and H⁺ Secretion. *As Pco₂ increases, the amount of H⁺ secreted increases. The elevated CO₂ in the renal tubular cell drives the reaction $CO_2 + H_2O \rightarrow H^+ + HCO_3^-$ to the right and subsequently increases H⁺ secretion.*

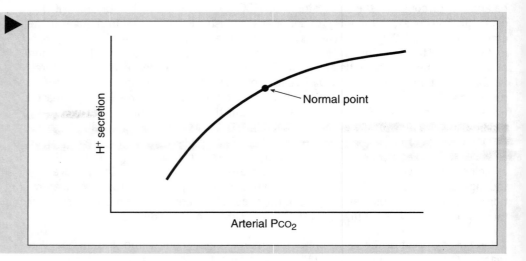

Aldosterone increases tubular H⁺ secretion and HCO₃⁻ generation by stimulating H⁺-ATPase in the intercalated cells of the collecting tubule system.

Aldosterone. In addition to its effect on Na⁺ and K⁺ transport, aldosterone stimulates H⁺ secretion. The overall mechanism of action of aldosterone is shown in Fig. 7-9. Besides increasing the apical membrane permeability to Na⁺ and K⁺ and stimulating the Na⁺–K⁺-ATPase in the principal cells, aldosterone stimulates a H⁺-ATPase in the intercalated cells of the collecting tubule system and increases H⁺ secretion. H⁺ per se has no effect on aldosterone secretion by the adrenal gland. However, stimuli that directly increase aldosterone secretion, such as extracellular volume contraction or elevated angiotensin II, may result in increased H⁺ secretion and a resulting systemic alkalosis.

Proximal Tubule Sodium Reabsorption. At first it may seem illogical to equate proximal tubule Na⁺ reabsorption with alterations in H⁺ secretion by the kidney. However, recall that a large portion of the Na⁺ reabsorbed in the proximal tubule occurs at the apical membrane in exchange for a secreted H⁺. Thus any stimulus that increases or decreases

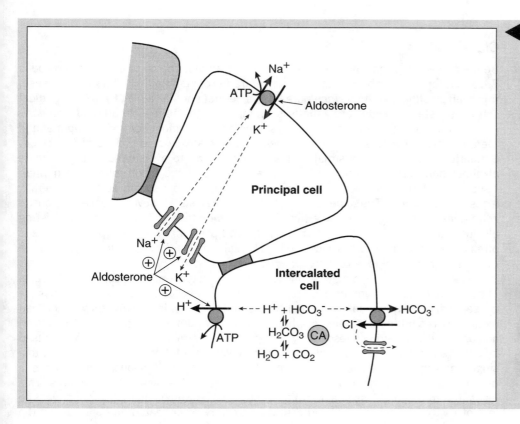

FIGURE 7-9
Mechanism of Aldosterone Modulation of H+ Secretion in Renal Tubule Cell. *In addition to stimulating Na+ reabsorption in the principal cells, aldosterone also stimulates H+-ATPase in the intercalated cells, resulting in increased H+ secretion. CA = carbonic anhydrase.*

proximal tubular Na^+ reabsorption may also increase or decrease H^+ secretion in the proximal tubule. For instance, loss of extracellular volume, which might occur during dehydration, increases the plasma protein concentration and elevates the colloid osmotic pressure. At the level of the peritubular capillary, the increased colloid osmotic pressure leads to increased Na^+ reabsorption and increased H^+ secretion. Conversely, factors that decrease Na^+ reabsorption also decrease H^+ secretion by the proximal tubule.

Plasma H+ Concentration. In an acidosis there is an increased cellular H^+ concentration. In addition to stimulating the production of NH_4^+ by the proximal tubule and increasing NH_4^+ excretion by the kidney, increased H^+ in the intercalated cells also results in increased H^+ secretion. While the proximal tubule response to increase NH_4^+ production requires a considerable period of time (hours to days), the increase in H^+ secretion occurs rapidly. The simplest proposed mechanism for the increased H^+ secretion is an increase in the supply of H^+ to the H^+-ATPase. Increasing or decreasing H^+ availability to the pump increases or decreases H^+ secretion.

> *Increased proximal tubule Na^+ reabsorption increases tubular H^+ secretion and HCO_3^- generation.*

> *Increased plasma H^+ concentration increases tubular H^+ secretion and HCO_3^- generation.*

ACID-BASE IMBALANCE

Normal plasma H^+ concentration or pH depends on the integrated balance of the three systems involved in acid–base balance. Any situation that impinges on any one of the three systems can alter the acid–base status of the body. For instance, loss of HCO_3^- as a result of diarrhea may severely impair the ability of the body to buffer free H^+, and elimination of CO_2 is many times decreased in patients with pulmonary disease. Many fluid and electrolyte disturbances alter renal function, which in turn affects the renal handling of H^+. Recognition of the interplay and actions of the buffers, the lungs, and the kidneys is necessary to understand fully the regulation of H^+ balance.

Classification

Before proceeding, some nomenclature must be clarified. The normal pH of the blood is 7.4 and is represented by a plasma H$^+$ concentration of 40 nmol/L. In the strictest sense, this is an alkaline condition since pure H$_2$O is neutral and has a pH of 7.0. In a clinical setting, the state of acidity or alkalinity is referenced to the normal condition. An *acidosis* is a situation that tends to result in a systemic condition more acidic than normal and therefore has a pH less than 7.4; *acidemia* is a relatively acidic state of the blood. Similarly, an *alkalosis* is a situation that tends to lead to a systemic condition more alkaline than normal; *alkalemia* is an alkaline state of the blood relative to normal. Usually, the terms are used interchangeably and justifiably so. An acidosis generally leads to an acidemia. The same logic applies to an alkalosis. However, equal and opposite conditions may exist at the same time. Thus, it is quite possible to have a coexisting alkalosis and acidosis that lead to a normal blood pH. Finally, a description of state is often used. A patient who has a low blood pH is said to be *acidotic*, while one with a high pH relative to normal is said to be *alkalotic*.

Acid–base imbalance may be divided into four categories of condition and cause. The first two categories are the conditions of acidosis and alkalosis. If the condition is the consequence of a pulmonary abnormality, it is said to be respiratory. Anything other than respiratory is said to be metabolic, which may be any number of situations. There is an acidosis caused by either a respiratory or metabolic abnormality, and an alkalosis caused by either a respiratory or metabolic abnormality. Most acid–base disturbances fit into a single category; however, several combinations can exist simultaneously. For instance, a person with emphysema and CO$_2$ retention may contract a gastrointestinal virus. This leads to vomiting and loss of acid from the stomach as well as diarrhea, which leads to loss of HCO$_3^-$ in the stool. Mixed disorders are very complicated and are beyond the scope of this book. However, recognition of the cause and compensation for each single disorder is a good place to start.

	Condition	
	Acidosis	**Alkalosis**
Cause	Respiratory	Respiratory
	Metabolic	Metabolic

Cause and Compensation

The relationship between a primary change in acid–base status and the resulting compensation is shown in Fig. 7-10. A disturbance in respiratory function that results in a change in arterial Pco$_2$, brings about a change in the plasma H$^+$ concentration and an appropriate renal compensation. For example, the renal response to an increase in arterial Pco$_2$ is to increase H$^+$ secretion and HCO$_3^-$ generation. The increase in plasma HCO$_3^-$ concentration returns the plasma H$^+$ concentration toward normal (Fig. 7-10A). A similar relationship between primary changes in plasma HCO$_3^-$ concentration and the resulting respiratory compensation is shown in Fig. 7-10B. The change in plasma HCO$_3^-$ concentration results in changes in plasma H$^+$ concentration. The resulting change in plasma H$^+$ alters alveolar ventilation to change the arterial Pco$_2$ and return the plasma H$^+$ toward normal. Thus any acid–base change caused primarily by one system results in a compensation by the complementary system. Since there are only four possible single disorders, each can be analyzed independently.

A primary respiratory or metabolic acid–base disturbance results in an acid–base compensation by the complementary system to minimize the acid–base disturbance.

RESPIRATORY ACIDOSIS

The cause of a respiratory acidosis is an increase in the Pco$_2$ in the blood generally resulting from an inability of the lungs to excrete CO$_2$ properly. As can be seen from the Henderson equation below, the increased Pco$_2$ directly results in an increase in the plasma H$^+$ concentration.

$$\frac{\uparrow Pco_2}{HCO_3^-} \, K = \uparrow H^+$$

*A **respiratory acidosis** can be characterized by an increased arterial Pco$_2$ and a compensatory increase in plasma HCO$_3^-$ concentration.*

Thus we have the condition of acidosis, and the cause is respiratory in nature. The obvious compensation for the elevated CO$_2$ would be an increase in plasma HCO$_3^-$ to minimize the increase in plasma H$^+$ concentration.

The first thought one might have is that, of course, the HCO_3^- will increase since increased CO_2 will elevate the HCO_3^- because of the equilibrium between CO_2 and HCO_3^- discussed above.

$$\uparrow CO_2 + H_2O \rightarrow \uparrow HCO_3^- + H^+$$

The logic is correct. The HCO_3^- concentration is increased. However, a quantitative analysis shows that the increase in HCO_3^- is insignificant. Recall that the solubility of CO_2 in blood is only 0.03 mmol/L per mm Hg of pressure. If the Pco_2 were to double from a normal 40 mm Hg to 80 mm Hg, the resulting increase in Pco_2 of 40 mm Hg would only amount to an additional 1.2 mmol/L increase in HCO_3^- concentration (40 mm Hg × 0.03 mmol/L per mm Hg = 1.2 mmol/L). Assuming all of the CO_2 were converted to HCO_3^-, the HCO_3^- would only increase from the normal 24 mEq/L to 25.2 mEq/L. This represents a 5% increase in HCO_3^- to compensate for a 100% increase in Pco_2. The

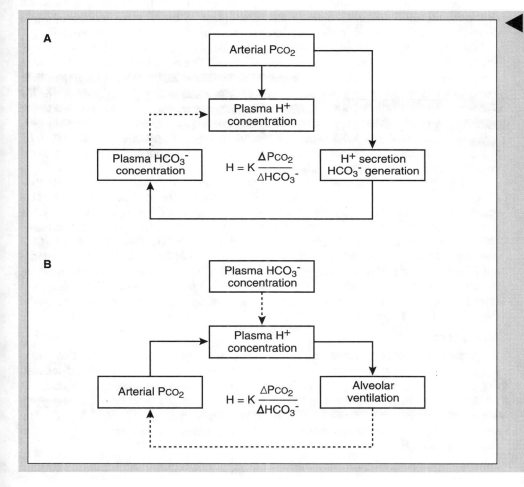

FIGURE 7-10
Relationship between Respiratory and Renal Systems in Regulation of Acid–Base Balance. (A) The compensation of the kidneys for a change in plasma H^+ concentration resulting from a primary respiratory change in arterial Pco_2 (ΔPco_2) is an appropriate change in plasma HCO_3^- (ΔHCO_3^-) to minimize the change in plasma H^+ concentration. (B) The compensation of the lungs for a change in plasma H^+ concentration resulting from a primary metabolic change in plasma HCO_3^- concentration (ΔHCO_3^-) is an appropriate change in arterial Pco_2 (ΔPco_2) to minimize the change in plasma H^+ concentration.

kidney must be called on to bring about a meaningful increase in plasma HCO_3^-. The increased Pco_2 acts as a stimulus to increase the formation of H^+ and HCO_3^- from CO_2 and H_2O in the renal tubular cells. The H^+ is secreted, and the new HCO_3^- is returned to the plasma to increase the plasma HCO_3^- concentration. The cause of the respiratory acidosis is CO_2 retention by the lungs. The increased Pco_2 results in a compensatory increase in plasma HCO_3^- by the kidney to minimize the change in plasma H^+ concentration.

It must be emphasized that the kidneys cannot *correct* the respiratory acidosis; they can only compensate for it. The reason is simple. The reaction between $CO_2 + H_2O$ and $H^+ + HCO_3^-$ is in equilibrium, depending on the relative concentrations of the components. At first the increased CO_2 forces the formation of $H^+ + HCO_3^-$ from CO_2 and H_2O. As the plasma and cell concentrations of HCO_3^- increase, the increased HCO_3^- concentration acts as a negative feedback and impedes the further formation of HCO_3^-. The renal cells arrive at a new equilibrium, with high CO_2 stimulating and increased HCO_3^- concentration inhibiting the rate of formation of additional HCO_3^-. The resulting plasma HCO_3^- concentration is simply insufficient to correct for the respiratory acidosis completely. One final and important point regarding compensation. Whether the primary cause is a respiratory or metabolic acid–base disorder, the disturbance results in a secondary compensation; the compensation returns the H^+ toward normal, but it can never fully correct the change in H^+ concentration resulting from the primary abnormality.

RESPIRATORY ALKALOSIS

> A **respiratory alkalosis** can be characterized by a decreased arterial Pco_2 and a compensatory decrease in plasma HCO_3^- concentration.

In most ways a respiratory alkalosis and the resulting renal compensation are mirror images of respiratory acidosis. The primary disturbance is a decrease in arterial Pco_2 due to hyperventilation, which may result from any number of stimuli including respiratory responses to high altitude, neural infections, or psychological dyspnea. A quick perusal of the Henderson equation illustrates that a decrease in the arterial Pco_2 results in a decrease in the plasma H^+ concentration. Because of the equilibrium between $CO_2 + H_2O$ and $H^+ + HCO_3^-$, the decreased CO_2 leads to a small but insignificant decrease in HCO_3^-. As described above, renal function is altered. The renal compensation is again a function of the change in the Pco_2. The decreased CO_2 decreases the generation of H^+ and HCO_3^- from CO_2 and H_2O in the cells. The decreased H^+ and HCO_3^- result in a decrease in both the amount of H^+ secreted and the amount of HCO_3^- returned to the plasma. In addition to the decreased HCO_3^- generated, the decreased H^+ secretion results in decreased reabsorption of filtered HCO_3^- and a loss of HCO_3^- in the urine. All the above factors lead to a decrease in plasma HCO_3^- concentration and a renal compensation for the respiratory alkalosis.

Just as the kidneys compensate for but do not correct the change in H^+ concentration resulting from a respiratory acidosis, they compensate for but do not correct a respiratory alkalosis. At first, the decrease in CO_2 in the renal cells decreases the formation of H^+ and HCO_3^-, and the plasma HCO_3^- falls. However, the decreased HCO_3^- concentration tends to promote the formation of HCO_3^- from CO_2 and H_2O. A new equilibruim is reached, and the resulting plasma HCO_3^- is decreased but not sufficiently to completely correct for the decreased plasma H^+ concentration. However, the degree to which the kidneys alter plasma HCO_3^- in response to respiratory changes in arterial Pco_2 is so precise that the resulting plasma HCO_3^- can be accurately predicted if the arterial Pco_2 is known.

METABOLIC ACIDOSIS

Respiratory acid–base disturbances result from alterations in pulmonary function. However, metabolic disturbances can result for any number of reasons and some are discussed in a subsequent section (see Clinical Examples). Renal disease can result in acidosis, but most metabolic acid–base changes are not caused by impaired renal function. Metabolic changes in acid–base status involve alterations in plasma HCO_3^- concentration. The Henderson equation below illustrates the relationship between plasma HCO_3^- concentration and plasma H^+ concentration.

$$\frac{Pco_2}{HCO_3^-} K = H^+$$

> A **metabolic acidosis** can be characterized by a decreased plasma HCO_3^- and a compensatory decrease in arterial Pco_2.

It can easily be seen that any change in HCO_3^- will alter the H^+ concentration. Metabolic acidosis results from a decrease in HCO_3^- concentration, and a resulting increase in plasma H^+ concentration. While the renal compensation for a respiratory acidosis is slow to develop, the respiratory response to a metabolic acidosis is very rapid. Increased H^+ is a very potent stimulus to increase ventilation. The increased ventilation rapidly lowers the arterial Pco_2 and returns the H^+ concentration toward normal.

While the lungs can rapidly compensate for the metabolic acidosis, they cannot correct the H^+ imbalance. As shown in Fig. 7-4, both high Pco_2 and high H^+ (low pH) stimulate alveolar ventilation. In this case, the increased H^+ stimulates ventilation and lowers Pco_2. However, the resulting decrease in arterial Pco_2 inhibits respiration. The two signals compete at the respiratory center, and the net result is increased alveolar ventilation and a compensation for the metabolic acidosis. However, the increased ventilation is insufficient to return the plasma H+ concentration to normal and metabolic acidosis with respiratory compensation results.

METABOLIC ALKALOSIS

Metabolic alkalosis is the result of an increased plasma HCO_3^- concentration. The increased HCO_3^- results in a decreased plasma H+ concentration. The respiratory compensation for metabolic alkalosis is simply the reverse of the compensation for metabolic acidosis. Decreased plasma H+ concentration inhibits the respiratory drive to ventilate, and the Pco_2 increases. However, increased arterial Pco_2 is a very potent stimulus to increase ventilation and thus Pco_2 only slightly increases. Thus the respiratory compensation for metabolic alkalosis is not nearly so powerful as the respiratory compensation for metabolic acidosis. In severe cases of metabolic acidosis, the Pco_2 may fall to less than 20 mm Hg, while in metabolic alkalosis the Pco_2 may only increase by a few mm Hg. Nevertheless, the relationship between plasma HCO_3^- and Pco_2 is predictable; that is, if the plasma HCO_3^- is known, the Pco_2 can be accurately estimated.

*A **metabolic alkalosis** can be characterized by an increased plasma HCO_3^- concentration and a compensatory increase in arterial Pco_2.*

RENAL RESPONSE TO METABOLIC DISTURBANCES

It is easy to understand how a respiratory acid–base disturbance may be corrected. In a patient unable to excrete CO_2, the resulting respiratory acidosis may be corrected by resolving the cause of the CO_2 retention. Increasing the alveolar ventilation by mechanical means can be used to lower the Pco_2 to normal levels and obviate the acid condition. Similarly, hyperventilation and decreased Pco_2 may be corrected by resolving the cause of the hyperventilation. For instance, returning from high altitude to sea level, where Po_2 is normal, will remove the hypoxic respiratory drive to hyperventilate and eliminate the cause of the respiratory alkalosis.

In many metabolic disturbances it is not quite so easy to explain logically the resulting physiologic adjustments by the body. Consider, for instance, a metabolic acidosis resulting from the loss of HCO_3^- in the stool because of diarrhea. The respiratory compensation for a metabolic acidosis is hyperventilation and an appropriate decrease in the arterial Pco_2. The first need of the body is protection from a severe increase in plasma H+ concentration resulting from the loss of HCO_3^-. In a healthy individual, the respiratory system performs that function quite nicely. The second need of the body is the restoration of the plasma HCO_3^- concentration to normal. The simplest way to increase the body HCO_3^- stores is to increase HCO_3^- generation in the kidney. However, the major stimulus for HCO_3^- generation in the renal tubular cells is arterial Pco_2, but, because of the respiratory compensation, the Pco_2 is decreased. Where then is the stimulus for increased HCO_3^- generation?

Similar considerations apply to a metabolic alkalosis. Consider an otherwise healthy individual who contracts a stomach virus and vomits. Normally, the HCO_3^- generated in the stomach lining, when H+ is secreted into the stomach lumen, is secreted into the small intestine to neutralize the H+ when the stomach empties. However, the H+ and Cl- are lost to the environment in the vomitus, and the plasma HCO_3^- concentration increases. The lungs compensate for the resulting metabolic alkalosis, and the arterial Pco_2 increases. The appropriate renal response should be decreased HCO_3^- reabsorption and loss of HCO_3^- in the urine to lower the plasma HCO_3^- concentration. However, the increased Pco_2 is a stimulus to increase HCO_3^- reabsorption. How then does the kidney decrease HCO_3^- reabsorption in the face of an increased arterial Pco_2?

The answer to both questions lies in the quantitative relationship between the filtered load of HCO_3^- and the H+ secreted by the kidney. It can be shown in both metabolic acidosis and metabolic alkalosis that there is an advantageous physiologic mismatch between the amount of filtered HCO_3^- and the amount of H+ secreted, so that the plasma HCO_3^- concentration is eventually returned to normal levels. Recall that during the respiratory compensation for metabolic disturbances the relative change in arterial Pco_2 is less than the change in plasma HCO_3^- concentration. Thus the change in H+ secretion is less than the change in the filtered load of HCO_3^-.

The quantitative relationship between the filtered load of HCO_3^-, H+ secretion, and HCO_3^- gain for a 70-kg adult is shown in Table 7-2.

Many acute metabolic acid–base disturbances of a nonrenal origin can be corrected by a healthy kidney through renal changes in H+ excretion and HCO_3^- reabsorption.

TABLE 7-2 ▶
Renal Response to Metabolic Acidosis

	Filtration Rate (L/day)	Plasma HCO₃⁻ (mEq/L)	HCO₃⁻ Filtered (mEq/d)	Arterial Pco₂ (mm Hg)	H⁺ Secreted (mEq/d)	HCO₃⁻ Reabsorbed (mEq/d)	HCO₃⁻ Gain (mEq/d)
Normal	180	24	4320	40	4370	4320	50
Acidosis	180	12	2160	26	2310	2160	150

Under normal conditions, H⁺ secretion in the kidney is sufficient to reabsorb all the filtered HCO_3^- and return about 50 mEq of new HCO_3^- to the plasma as a result of the formation of titratable acids and NH_4^+. In the example given, the metabolic acidosis was severe enough to lower the plasma HCO_3^- by 50% to 12 mEq/L. Thus the filtered HCO_3^- decreased by 50%. The respiratory compensation was appropriate, and the hyperventilation decreased the Pco_2 by 40% to 26 mm Hg. The H⁺ secretion was appropriately decreased but relatively less than the filtered load of HCO_3^-. Therefore in the case of metabolic acidosis the H⁺ secretion is decreased, but it is still sufficient to reabsorb all the filtered HCO_3^- and increase the amount of new HCO_3^- returned to the plasma. It should be intuitive that the additional H⁺ secretion was used to form new titratable acids and, most probably, NH_4^+. Each titratable acid and NH_4^+ formed and excreted in the urine results in the addition of new HCO_3^- to the plasma.

The case for metabolic alkalosis is shown in Table 7-3.

TABLE 7-3 ▶
Renal Response to Metabolic Alkalosis

	Filtration Rate (L/day)	Plasma HCO₃⁻ (mEq/L)	HCO₃⁻ Filtered (mEq/d)	Arterial Pco₂ (mm Hg)	H⁺ Secreted (mEq/d)	HCO₃⁻ Reabsorbed (mEq/d)	HCO₃⁻ Gain (mEq/d)
Normal	180	24	4320	40	4370	4320	50
Alkalosis	180	37	6660	50	6530	6660	−130

In this situation, the metabolic alkalosis resulted from a plasma HCO_3^- increase to 37 mEq/L. The appropriate respiratory hypoventilation increased the arterial Pco_2 by 20% to 50 mm Hg. The H⁺ secretion increased, but the increase is inadequate to reabsorb all the additional filtered HCO_3^-. As a result, HCO_3^- will be lost in the urine, and plasma HCO_3^- concentration will decrease.

While it may seem illogical that with a metabolic acidosis a decrease in arterial Pco_2 will result in a net increase in plasma HCO_3^- concentration or that an increase in arterial Pco_2 will result in a net decrease in plasma HCO_3^- concentration during metabolic alkalosis, the effect of simultaneous changes in plasma HCO_3^- that occur must be considered. The mismatch between filtered HCO_3^- and H⁺ secretion is physiologically appropriate; it allows the kidneys to correct for nonrenal disturbances in metabolic acid–base disorders. It must be emphasized that the kidney is slow to respond. Any sustained disturbance will continue to result in the acid–base imbalance. Prolonged diarrhea, for instance, results in a continuous loss of HCO_3^- which occurs faster than the kidney can generate new HCO_3^-. Only when the diarrhea is stopped can the kidney correct the acid–base disturbance.

Diagnosis

Once the physiologic mechanisms of cause and compensation are understood it is a relatively simple matter to derive some guidelines in the diagnosis of single acid–base disorders (Table 7-4). It must be emphasized that multiple disorders can occur and thorough diagnosis of them is sometimes difficult if not almost impossible. The acid–base state is given for the arterial H⁺ concentration and pH as well as the ratio of the variables used in the Henderson-Hasselbalch equation.

	Pco_2	HCO_3^-	H^+	pH	$HCO_3^-/0.03 \times Pco_2$
Respiratory acidosis	↑	↑	> 45 nmol/L	< 7.35	< 20/1
Respiratory alkalosis	↓	↓	< 35 nmol/L	> 7.45	> 20/1
Metabolic acidosis	↓	↓	> 45 nmol/L	< 7.35	< 20/1
Metabolic alkalosis	↑	↑	< 35 nmol/L	> 7.45	> 20/1

TABLE 7-4
Summary of Primary Acid–Base Disturbances. The primary cause is given a bold arrow while the appropriate compensation has a lighter arrow.

The first consideration when making an acid–base disorder diagnosis is obviously to obtain the acid–base status. This can be determined by looking at the arterial H^+ concentration or the pH, whichever is available. There is a small range of normal values for both measurements. The arterial H^+ concentration normally varies between 35 and 45 nmol/L. Any value greater than 45 nmol/L is considered acidotic and any value less than 35 nmol/L is alkalotic. Similarly, the normal arterial pH varies between 7.35 and 7.45. Any value less than 7.35 is considered acidotic and any value greater than 7.45 is considered alkalotic.

The first step in the diagnosis of an acid–base disturbance is to determine the acid–base condition of the blood. The second step is to determine the cause of the acid–base disturbance.

Once the acid–base status has been determined, the second step is to identify the cause. As shown in Table 7-4, there are only two possibilities for acidosis. Either the arterial Pco_2 is elevated (respiratory acidosis) or the plasma HCO_3^- concentration is decreased (metabolic acidosis). There are no other possibilities. There are also only two possibilities for alkalosis. Either the arterial Pco_2 is decreased or the plasma HCO_3^- concentration is increased. If these two simple steps are followed, the diagnosis of acidosis or alkalosis can be determined to be of respiratory or metabolic origin.

A word of caution is in order. The compensatory changes are also shown in Table 7-4, and it is often tempting to look at something other than the acid–base status and attempt to make a diagnosis. For example, an elevated arterial Pco_2 may be interpreted as a respiratory acidosis when it is an appropriate compensation for metabolic alkalosis. Similarly, an increased plasma HCO_3^- concentration might be taken to indicate a metabolic alkalosis when it is actually the renal compensation for a respiratory acidosis, and so on for other combinations.

A definitive diagnosis can be made for any single acid–base disorder. However, there is often more than one underlying disorder. There are many rules of thumb that apply to established and stable single acid–base disorders. As pointed out above, the compensatory response to any single acid–base disorder is predictable. Empirical observations on large numbers of patients known to have only one acid–base disorder have been used to develop reasonable quantitative relationships between the change in the primary variable causing the disturbance and the change in the compensatory response. One set of these relationships is given in Table 7-5.

Condition	Primary Variable	Compensatory Response
Respiratory Acidosis	↑ Pco_2	↑ HCO_3^- (0.35 mEq/L per mm Hg ↑ Pco_2)
Respiratory Alkalosis	↓ Pco_2	↓ HCO_3^- (0.5 mEq/L per mm Hg ↓ Pco_2)
Metabolic Acidosis	↓ HCO_3^-	↓ Pco_2 (1.2 mm Hg per mEq/L ↓ HCO_3^-)
Metabolic Alkalosis	↑ HCO_3^-	↑ Pco_2 (0.6 mm Hg per mEq/L ↑ HCO_3^-)

TABLE 7-5
Quantitative Relationships between the Change in the Primary Variable and the Change in the Compensatory Response

The relationships given are only one set of many in general use and are reasonably accurate. In established acid–base disorders they can be used with a good medical history to determine if only a single disorder is present. For instance, in established respiratory acidosis each 1 mm Hg increase in arterial Pco_2 should result in a compensatory increase in plasma HCO_3^- of 0.35 mEq/L. In an otherwise healthy individual with chronic respiratory acidosis, an increase in arterial Pco_2 from 40 to 70 mm Hg results in an increase in plasma HCO_3^- of about 10.5 mEq/L. The plasma HCO_3^- concentration thus increases from the normal 24 mEq/L to 34.5 mEq/L as a result of renal compensation. Similarly, in simple metabolic acidosis a 1 mEq/L decrease in HCO_3^- should result in a 1.2 mm Hg decrease in arterial Pco_2. If the patient's blood gas measurements agree with the predicted changes, a single disorder is most likely. If they do not, more than one disorder should be suspected.

Clinical Examples

Acid–base disorders can occur for a variety of reasons. Clinical examples perhaps best illustrate these disturbances and provide some additional understanding of the normal maintenance of acid–base balance. Before proceeding, it is necessary to understand that any acid–base disturbance must have a cause and that the cause must be sustained. Holding one's breath results in an acute respiratory acidosis, but only transiently until normal breathing is resumed. However, a prolonged inability to exhale CO_2 results in a sustained respiratory acidosis and produces a stable but predictable outcome. Likewise, short-term strenuous exercise may result in a metabolic lactic acidosis that will resolve upon cessation of the exercise. However, a long-term acid insult may result in sustained metabolic acidosis. The clinical case given at the beginning of the chapter is another such example.

RESPIRATORY ACIDOSIS

An anxious, 20-year-old asthmatic woman presented in the emergency room with a respiratory rate greater than 30 breaths/min and wheezing. An arterial blood gas analysis gave the following results: Po_2, 60 mm Hg; Pco_2, 56 mm Hg; pH/H+, 7.29/51 nmol/L; and HCO_3^-, 27 mEq/L.

This patient has two obvious problems. The first is hypoxia, since the Po_2 is markedly depressed compared to the normal 100 mm Hg. The second is an acid–base disorder. She is acidotic since both the pH and the H+ concentrations indicate an acidemia. It is a respiratory acidosis because the arterial Pco_2 is elevated. There is renal compensation since the plasma HCO_3^- concentration is mildly elevated. If the cause of the acidosis were metabolic in nature, the plasma HCO_3^- would have been depressed.

The most serious condition in this patient is the severe hypoxia, which can be life-threatening. In many instances pulmonary dysfunction presents a more serious concern with O_2 uptake than with CO_2 retention. This is particularly true with gas diffusion disturbances such as pneumonia. The solubility of CO_2 in body fluids is much greater than O_2; therefore, the inability to exchange O_2 from the alveolae to the blood is often greatly reduced with pulmonary congestion before any impediment to CO_2 exchange occurs. Often the increased respiratory drive that occurs with hypoxia results in an actual decrease in Pco_2 and a respiratory alkalosis, even though O_2 uptake in the lungs is reduced. In fact, in the case presented the marked respiratory drive as a result of the reduced Po_2 as well as the increased H+ concentration may have prevented a more severe CO_2 retention and increased acidosis. This patient was eventually diagnosed as having severe bronchoconstriction of several days duration. Thus the cause of the acid–base abnormality is an inability to excrete CO_2 because of an increased resistance to alveolar ventilation that persisted over several days.

RESPIRATORY ALKALOSIS

A patient with severe muscular weakness resulting from myasthenia gravis was ventilated with a constant-volume respirator. At 1 hour, his arterial blood showed: Po_2, 100 mm Hg; Pco_2, 25 mm Hg; pH/H+, 7.60/24.5 nmol/L; and HCO_3^-, 24.5 mEq/L. At 2 days, his arterial blood showed: Po_2, 100 mm Hg; Pco_2, 25 mm Hg; pH/H+, 7.47/32.4 nmol/L; and HCO_3^-, 18.5 mEq/L.

To appreciate the time course of the renal compensation for respiratory dysfunction in this case, an acid–base diagnosis must be made at two different time points. As discussed in the case above on respiratory acidosis, many respiratory problems result in difficulty with O_2 uptake before problems with CO_2 retention occur. Although no data are available for pretreatment Po_2 levels, the patient was undoubtedly placed on the respirator to correct a hypoxic condition because of severe muscular weakness and the inability to regulate O_2 uptake properly. However, at 1 hour it can be seen that the degree of ventilation was in excess of that necessary to regulate the arterial Pco_2, and it is decreased. The resulting condition is a marked alkalosis as evidenced by the increased pH and decreased H^+ concentration. Thus the diagnosis of respiratory alkalosis can be made. However, the HCO_3^- concentration is almost exactly normal. Does this indicate that there is renal involvement? No, the kidney simply has not had the appropriate time for compensation. While the pulmonary system may alter the Pco_2 in a matter of a few minutes, the kidneys may take several hours or even days to compensate for respiratory disturbances completely.

The information necessary to make an acid–base diagnosis after 2 days on the respirator is also given. The respiratory alkalosis is still present, but it is much less severe in spite of the fact that the Pco_2 has not changed. The reason is that the kidneys have had sufficient time to compensate for the respiratory dysfunction. Over the course of the 2 days, the plasma HCO_3^- has fallen from a near normal value to 18.5 mEq/L, and the patient has gone from a simple acute respiratory alkalosis to a stable condition of respiratory alkalosis with renal compensation. The cause of the alkalosis is hyperventilation induced by mechanical means over the 2-day course of the treatment.

An understanding of the time course of the renal compensation for respiratory alkalosis is germane to this patient's treatment. If the patient is removed from the respirator, the Pco_2 will increase. Because of renal compensation, the blood pH is near normal, and an increase in Pco_2 to normal will result in an acidosis, since the HCO_3^- concentration is low. If blood gases are obtained shortly after the cessation of treatment, the blood gas analysis would indicate an acidosis. Without an understanding of the time required for renal compensation, it might be assumed that the acidosis is a result of CO_2 retention. It would be a mistake to place the patient back on the respirator and lower the Pco_2 to correct the acidosis. It is simply unnecessary. The much more prudent action would be to leave the patient alone and give the kidneys time to increase the HCO_3^- concentration to the appropriate level.

METABOLIC ACIDOSIS

A 58-year-old man developed severe diarrhea. The volume of diarrheal fluid was approximately 1 L/hr. Pertinent laboratory data include: Na^+, 138 mEq/L; K^+, 3.8 mEq/L; Cl^-, 120 mEq/L; HCO_3^-, 9 mEq/L; pH 7.2/H^+, 59.0 nmol/L; and Pco_2, 22 mm Hg.

This patient has an acidemic condition in the blood and is therefore acidotic. The cause of the acidosis is metabolic since the HCO_3^- concentration is low. If the cause of the acidosis were respiratory, the Pco_2 would be elevated, but it is low. Therefore, the patient has a metabolic acidosis with respiratory compensation. The cause of the metabolic acidosis may not be intuitively obvious. It is the loss of HCO_3^- in the diarrheal fluid that is responsible for the decreased HCO_3^- in the plasma. In the stomach wall, CO_2 and H_2O combine to form H^+ and HCO_3^-. The H^+ is secreted into the lumen of the stomach in exchange for K^+. HCO_3^- is secreted into the pancreatic ducts in exchange for Cl^-. The HCO_3^- concentration in pancreatic secretions can reach very high levels. Normally, the pancreatic secretions are used to neutralize the H^+ in the stomach contents when the stomach empties. However, periods of excessively increased intestinal motility, which occur during diarrhea, result in the movement of the HCO_3^- down the intestines and the loss of HCO_3^- in the stool. The cause of the sustained acidosis is this sustained loss of HCO_3^-. The kidneys reabsorb all of the filtered HCO_3^- in addition to generating new HCO_3^-. However, the loss of HCO_3^- in the diarrheal fluid is so great in this patient that the kidneys cannot manufacture enough new HCO_3^- to keep up with the loss. If the cause of the diarrhea is controlled and the fluid replaced, the kidneys can eventually make enough HCO_3^- to replace the body stores. Additional HCO_3^- is unnecessary to correct the acidotic condition, but it may be given.

The plasma Na^+ concentration is normal despite the loss of a rather large volume of fluid from the body, and the patient is undoubtedly volume contracted. As discussed in previous chapters, Na^+ is the major determinant of extracellular volume. All of the Na^+ conserving mechanisms are activated, and there is avid Na^+ reabsorption by the kidneys.

Antidiuretic hormone (ADH) is also elevated, and H_2O is conserved by the kidney to maintain normal plasma osmolarity. The Cl^- concentration is elevated. Since the secretion of HCO_3^- in the pancreas occurred in exchange for Cl^-, there is a gain of Cl^- concomitant with the lost HCO_3^-, and the plasma Cl^- concentration increased to maintain electroneutrality.

METABOLIC ALKALOSIS

A patient with a known duodenal ulcer had been vomiting for 3 weeks. The relevant data include: pH 7.55/H^+ 32.4 nmol/L; Pco_2, 50 mm Hg; HCO_3^-, 37 mEq/L; Na^+, 138 mEq/L; K^+, 2.4 mEq/L; and Cl^-, 85 mEq/L.

It can be determined from the blood chemistries that this patient is alkalotic since the blood pH is high and the H^+ concentration is low. The cause of the alkalosis is metabolic because the plasma HCO_3^- concentration is high. If the alkalosis were respiratory in nature, the Pco_2 would be low, but it too is slightly elevated, which is the appropriate compensation for metabolic alkalosis. Thus the full diagnosis is metabolic alkalosis with respiratory compensation.

The next most important step is the determination of the cause of the sustained alkalosis. The patient has lost volume and hydrochloric acid (HCl) from the stomach because of the vomiting. As a result of the loss of Cl^- and volume, the plasma HCO_3^- concentration is increased. However, the arterial Pco_2 is only marginally elevated. Since the increased Pco_2 stimulus to increase H^+ secretion and HCO_3^- reabsorption is weak, why is HCO_3^- not lost in the urine? In addition to the elevated arterial Pco_2, there are at least two mechanisms that keep the plasma HCO_3^- concentration high, and they are both related to the volume. One mechanism by which the kidney reacts to volume depletion is to increase proximal tubule reabsorption. Since the proximal tubule is the major site of HCO_3^- reabsorption, an increase in proximal reabsorption will also lead to increased HCO_3^- reabsorption. A second and probably more important mechanism is related to the renin–angiotensin–aldosterone system. A decrease in the effective circulating volume leads to activation of the renin–angiotensin system and a subsequent increase in plasma aldosterone concentration. In addition to its Na^+-retaining effect, aldosterone also increases H^+ secretion in the distal nephron. For every H^+ secreted in the kidney, a HCO_3^- is added to the body. The elevated Pco_2, increased proximal tubule reabsorption and elevated aldosterone combine to keep the plasma HCO_3^- concentration elevated.

At first it might seem counterproductive for the increased proximal tubule reabsorption and increased aldosterone to sustain a metabolic alkalosis. However, maintenance of the effective circulating volume takes priority over almost all other functions of the kidney. The body will go to great lengths to maintain volume even at the expense of acid–base status. In fact, the resolution of the alkalotic condition is rather simple. If the vomiting can be stopped and the patient given some saltwater to drink to replace the volume, the situation corrects itself. Restoration of the ECV will return the proximal tubule reabsorption to normal and also return plasma aldosterone concentration to normal, both of which will allow the filtered HCO_3^- to escape reabsorption. As HCO_3^- is lost in the urine, the plasma HCO_3^- concentration returns to normal. Without concomitant volume contraction, it is almost impossible to induce metabolic alkalosis by the ingestion of HCO_3^- because the filtered HCO_3^- will simply be excreted.

MIXED DISORDER

A 58-year-old man with a history of chronic bronchitis develops a severe case of diarrhea. He is admitted to the emergency room where his blood pressure is 105 mm Hg systolic and 65 mm Hg diastolic. His respiratory rate is 32 breaths/min. His laboratory data include: HCO_3^-, 9 mEq/L; Cl^-, 120 mEq/L; Na^+, 138 mEq/L; K^+, 3.2 mEq/L; pH, 6.79/H^+, 108 nmol/L; and Pco_2, 40 mm Hg.

On the surface this patient is very similar to the patient above with metabolic acidosis. In fact, all of the plasma values are the same except for the severe acidosis and the normal arterial Pco_2. The acidosis is severe enough to be imminently life-threatening. There is a metabolic component to the acidosis since the plasma HCO_3^- concentration is decreased. If the respiratory system were functioning normally, the increased respiratory rate surely would result in a decreased arterial Pco_2 to compensate for the metabolic disturbance. However, because of the bronchitis the patient is simply unable to exchange air and decrease the Pco_2. In spite of the hyperventilation, he is unable to lower the arterial Pco_2 below normal.

Because of the chronic nature of the bronchitis, it is likely that the patient had a preexisting respiratory acidosis that was compounded by the acute onset of the metabolic acidosis. In this case, heroic measures should be taken to save the patient's life. An infusion of HCO_3^- in an attempt to correct the acidosis is warranted until one of the conditions causing the acidosis can be alleviated.

RESOLUTION OF CLINICAL CASE

Any good, in-depth diagnosis takes into account all available information, including the patient history. There were two known possible abnormalities. First, the patient was a known diabetic and had a recent history of pneumonia. Both prior conditions pointed to a potential problem with acid–base disorders. He was confused, which suggested some interference with neurologic function. His respiratory rate was high, which indicated a pulmonary problem. Finally, the blood pressure was low, which suggested volume depletion. Given this history, it was necessary to look at the laboratory values for some additional help.

The two most striking abnormalities were the acidic condition of the plasma and the markedly elevated plasma glucose concentration. The patient was acidotic. Since there was a potential respiratory and a potential metabolic problem, the cause of the acidosis had to be determined. The plasma HCO_3^- concentration was decreased, which indicated a metabolic acidosis. Because the patient had a history of pneumonia, it was wise to determine if there was any respiratory involvement. Recall that during a metabolic acidosis the change in arterial Pco_2 can be predicted from the change in plasma HCO_3^- concentration if the respiratory system is functionally normal. For every 1 mEq/L change in plasma HCO_3^-, the Pco_2 should decrease by 1.2 mm Hg. Since the plasma HCO_3^- was decreased from the normal 24 mEq/L by 16 mEq/L, the predicted Pco_2 should have been decreased from the normal 40 mm Hg by about 19 mm Hg to a value of 21 mm Hg. The measured value for arterial Pco_2 of 20 mm Hg was very close to the predicted value. The conclusion drawn was that the acid–base disorder was a metabolic acidosis with appropriate respiratory compensation. If the history of pneumonia was of any consequence, it was not important in the pulmonary exchange of CO_2. The elevated plasma H^+ concentration was responsible for the increased respiratory rate and subsequent decrease in arterial Pco_2.

The plasma glucose concentration was the key to the cause of the metabolic acidosis. Normal plasma glucose concentration is usually less than 100 mg/dL. The patient had a markedly elevated plasma glucose concentration of 800 mg/dL. The patient was undoubtedly unable to metabolize glucose normally, probably because of a lack of insulin, and the plasma glucose concentration had increased. The inability to metabolize glucose means that the body must use protein and fats to sustain metabolism. The result is the generation of organic acids such as acetoacetic acid and β-hydroxybutyric acid. Since these acids are buffered by HCO_3^- in the plasma, the HCO_3^- concentration must decrease. The acidotic condition will stimulate the kidney to increase the production of NH_4^+ and increase the generation of new HCO_3^-, but the continued production of organic acids by the body will neutralize the new HCO_3^- produced and keep the plasma HCO_3^- concentration low.

The patient's blood pressure was low, an indirect indication of a low ECV, but the urine output was increased. When the ECV is low, the cause of the increased urine output must be diagnosed. Not only is glucose involved in the generation of the acidosis, it is also the cause of the increased urine output. The elevated plasma glucose concentration results in an increase in the filtered load of glucose. Since the plasma glucose concentration was very high, the amount of filtered glucose exceeded the ability of the proximal tubule to reabsorb glucose, and the tubular maximum for glucose was exceeded. Excess glucose in the tubular fluid acts as an osmotic particle and prevents normal H_2O

reabsorption. The decreased H_2O reabsorption naturally results in an increase in urine output. Thus, in this situation glucose acted as an osmotic diuretic.

Several additional values in the chemistry 7 panel that were obtained on the venous blood sample were germane to the condition and diagnosis of this patient. First the plasma creatinine and the BUN concentrations were within the normal range of values. Thus GFR appeared to be normal. However, the plasma Na^+ concentration was low, and the plasma K^+ concentration was increased. Finally, the anion gap—the calculated difference between the plasma Na^+ concentration and the measured Cl^- and HCO_3^- anion concentration—was increased relative to normal. All of these observations deserve consideration.

The key to the decreased plasma Na^+ concentration can be found in the plasma glucose concentration. Insulin promotes the movement of glucose into the cells. The lack of insulin in this patient resulted in an increase in extracellular glucose concentration. Increased extracellular glucose acts as an osmotic particle and causes the movement of H_2O out of the cells because of the increased extracellular osmolarity. The decreased plasma Na^+ concentration was the result of movement of H_2O into the extracellular space and subsequent dilution of the extracellular Na^+. Some of the confusion seen in the patient may well have resulted from intracellular dehydration of the cells in the central nervous system. If glucose is considered, the extracellular osmolarity is actually increased and illustrates one of the few times that plasma Na^+ concentration is not an accurate estimation of plasma osmolarity. If glucose is removed from the ECF, H_2O will move back into the cells, and the plasma Na^+ concentration will increase.

The plasma K^+ was increased. Because of the acidosis, the increased H^+ exchanges with K^+ in the cells and the extracellular K^+ concentration was increased. Although the plasma K^+ concentration was increased, the patient was probably K^+ depleted. One of the major factors that increase K^+ secretion by the kidney is an increase in the tubule fluid flow rate. As a result of the osmotic diuresis, the tubule fluid flow is increased in all segments of the nephron, and K^+ is washed out in the urine. The osmotic diuresis also resulted in volume depletion and stimulation of the renin–angiotensin–aldosterone system. A major action of aldosterone is to increase K^+ secretion and further increase K^+ loss from the body. Because of increased loss of K^+ in the urine, the patient's total body K^+ was certainly decreased in spite of the measured increase in plasma K^+ concentration. This presented the physician with a dilemma. The obvious treatment for this patient was to restore normal glucose metabolism with insulin treatment. However, if the treatment is too aggressive, the plasma glucose will be metabolized, and the resulting decrease in plasma H^+ concentration will promote the movement of K^+ into the cells, which are K^+ depleted. Insulin also promotes the cellular uptake of K^+. Both factors may result in a precipitous fall in plasma K^+ concentration and a threatening hypokalemia. The patient was volume depleted and required fluid replacement. The prudent course of action was to give the insulin in small doses over several hours and include K^+ in the intravenous fluid. It is very disconcerting to consider infusing K^+ into a patient with a preexisting hyperkalemia, and both the plasma K^+ and glucose concentrations should be monitored frequently.

Before closing, some mention should be made of the "anion gap." The anion gap is nothing more than the concentration differences between the major cation, Na^+, and the two major anions, Cl^- and HCO_3^-. In a normal individual, it typically ranges between 10–16 mEq with the Na^+ concentration greater than the sum of the Cl^- and HCO_3^- concentrations. This does not mean that plasma is not electrically neutral. The anions are there, but they are simply not measured during a routine chemical analysis of the plasma. A definitive acid–base diagnosis can only be made from an arterial blood sample. However, a rather good estimate of HCO_3^- can be obtained from a venous blood sample. In practice, a measured volume of plasma is exposed to a known P_{CO_2} and H^+ is added. The HCO_3^- combines with the H^+, and CO_2 is liberated from the reaction. Because about 95% of the liberated CO_2 comes from the HCO_3^- in the plasma, the amount of CO_2 liberated is a good estimate of the HCO_3^- concentration. This value is often referred to as total CO_2 or HCO_3^- (estimated) in laboratory reports. Deviation of the HCO_3^- concentration from normal is a first indication of some sort of acid–base abnormality whether it be metabolic or respiratory. If a subsequent arterial blood gas analysis indicates a metabolic acidosis, the anion gap can be put to good use in determining the cause of the acidosis. In the metabolic acidosis clinical example discussed earlier, the plasma HCO_3^- concentration was decreased as a result of loss of HCO_3^- in the stool, but the loss of the HCO_3^- anion was accompanied by an increase in the plasma Cl^- concentration. The anion gap $(Na^+-Cl^--HCO_3^-)$ was 9 mEq/L and essentially normal. The plasma HCO_3^- concentration in this case was also low. It had been consumed in the buffering of the organic acids in the plasma. The anions of the buffered organic acids replaced the HCO_3^- anion. In this case, the anion gap increased to 24 mEq/L. A history is frequently difficult to obtain in an emergency situation. The anion gap can be used to differentiate between a metabolic acidosis resulting from the loss of HCO_3^- from the body, as in severe diarrhea, or the addition of H^+ to the body, which could occur with ingestion of excess aspirin by a child.

REVIEW QUESTIONS

1. A patient with severe anemia might be expected to have

    (A) a decreased arterial P_{O_2}

    (B) a decreased arterial P_{CO_2}

    (C) a decreased venous pH

    (D) a decreased respiratory rate

2. The pK of any buffer solution is the pH at which the buffer pair concentrations are equal. For the $H_2PO_4^-$–HPO_4^{2-} buffer system the pK is 6.8. If 10 mEq of $H_2PO_4^-$ and 10 mEq of HPO_4^{2-} are added to a $NaHCO_3$ solution with a pH of 6.8, you would predict that the

    (A) pK of the $H_2PO_4^-$–HPO_4^{2-} buffer system will increase

    (B) pH of the solution will increase

    (C) HPO_4^{2-} concentration will increase relative to the $H_2PO_4^-$ concentration

    (D) buffering capacity of the solution will increase

3. Which of the following combinations of arterial blood conditions leads to the largest increase in alveolar ventilation?

    (A) Decreased pH and decreased P_{CO_2}

    (B) Decreased pH and increased P_{CO_2}

    (C) Increased pH and decreased P_{CO_2}

    (D) Increased pH and increased P_{CO_2}

4. Which of the following conditions increases the amount of H^+ secreted by the kidney?

    (A) Metabolic acidosis

    (B) Hyperventilation

    (C) Volume depletion

    (D) Respiratory alkalosis

5. Urinary excretion of NH_4^+ is increased by

    (A) increased proximal tubule reabsorption

    (B) increased plasma aldosterone concentration

    (C) increased plasma H^+ concentration

    (D) increased filtered HCO_3^-

6. An elderly patient on diuretic treatment for many years to control hypertension complains of weakness. He otherwise appears healthy. Routine analysis of a venous plasma sample gives two pertinent values. The estimated plasma HCO_3^- is 30 mmol/L, and the plasma K^+ is 2.5 mEq/L. It is likely that this patient has

    (A) a metabolic compensation for respiratory alkalosis resulting from anxiety-induced hyperventilation

    (B) a metabolic compensation for respiratory acidosis resulting from long-term cigarette smoking

    (C) a metabolic acidosis resulting from a recent case of diarrhea

    (D) a metabolic alkalosis resulting from long-term diuretic use

7. An unconscious patient is brought into the emergency room. The only available acid–base data are: arterial Pco_2, 20 mm Hg; and plasma HCO_3^-, 8 mEq/L. The acid–base diagnosis is

   (A) respiratory acidosis with metabolic compensation

   (B) respiratory alkalosis with metabolic compensation

   (C) metabolic acidosis with respiratory compensation

   (D) metabolic alkalosis with respiratory compensation

8. A very young patient has the following laboratory data: Pco_2, 26 mm Hg; HCO_3^-, 12 mEq/L; and H^+, 52 nmol/L. The anion gap ($Na^+ - Cl^- - HCO_3^-$) is 26 mEq/L. The most likely acid–base disorder is

   (A) respiratory acidosis due to broncoconstriction

   (B) respiratory acidosis due to an alveolar diffusion barrier

   (C) metabolic acidosis due to acid ingestion

   (D) metabolic acidosis due to loss of HCO_3^-

9. A patient has the following arterial blood gas data: Po_2, 95 mm Hg; Pco_2, 24 mm Hg; pH, 7.20; and HCO_3^-, 10 mEq/L.

   (A) respiratory acidosis with renal compensation

   (B) respiratory alkalosis with renal compensation

   (C) metabolic acidosis with respiratory compensation

   (D) metabolic alkalosis with respiratory compensation

10. A comatose patient is brought into the emergency room with a very high respiratory rate. His blood gases are: Pco_2, 45 mm Hg; HCO_3^-, 10 mEq/L; and pH, 6.94. The most likely disorder is

   (A) metabolic acidosis and respiratory alkalosis

   (B) metabolic alkalosis and respiratory acidosis

   (C) metabolic acidosis and respiratory acidosis

   (D) metabolic acidosis and respiratory alkalosis

11. The following laboratory data are obtained from a patient: pH/H^+, 7.24/58 nmol/L; Pco_2, 24 mm Hg; HCO_3^-, 10 mEq/L; Na^+, 135 mEq/L; K^+, 6.1 mEq/L; Cl^-, 90 mEq/L; and creatinine, 6 mg/dL. The patient has

   (A) respiratory alkalosis due to hyperventilation

   (B) metabolic acidosis due to loss of HCO_3^- during diarrhea

   (C) metabolic acidosis due to ingested acids

   (D) metabolic acidosis due to renal disease

ANSWERS AND EXPLANATIONS

1. **The answer is C.** A decreased amount of hemoglobin in the blood would decrease the amount of H^+ from the tissues that can be buffered by the red blood cells. Therefore the pH in the venous blood would decrease. Even though the hemoglobin concentration in the blood is decreased, the arterial Po_2 in the arterial blood would be normal. In the lungs the hemoglobin would be saturated. Even though the amount of O_2 carried in the blood would be decreased, the Po_2 would be normal. The CO_2 in the blood would also equilibrate with the alveolar gas, and the arterial Pco_2 would be

normal. If the decreased venous pH is still present in the arterial blood, the respiratory center is stimulated, and the respiratory rate increases, not decreases.

2. **The answer is D.** The ability of the solution to accept or donate H^+ increases because of the addition of the extra buffer pair. The pK is a fixed physical-chemical property of the buffer system. It is different for each different buffer pair but does not change for any individual buffer pair. Since the pH of the solution is the same as the pK of the $H_2PO_4^-$–HPO_4^{2-} system, neither the pH nor the relative concentration of $H_2PO_4^-$ and HPO_4^{2-} will change.

3. **The answer is B.** Both increased H^+ concentration (decreased pH) and increased P_{CO_2} in the arterial blood stimulates respiration, and they are additive. Increased pH and decreased arterial P_{CO_2} both inhibit respiration. The other two combinations tend to cancel each other.

4. **The answer is C.** Volume depletion leads to two physiologic responses that increase H^+ secretion by the kidney. First, the volume depletion leads to increased proximal tubule reabsorption. Since some of the Na^+ is reabsorbed in exchange for H^+, anything that increases Na^+ reabsorption also increases H^+ secretion. Second, and most important, volume depletion activates the renin–angiotensin–aldosterone system. Aldosterone stimulates the H^+-ATPase in the intercalated cells of the collecting duct to increase H^+ secretion. Metabolic acidosis leads to a respiratory compensation and a decreased P_{CO_2}. Decreased P_{CO_2} decreases H^+ secretion. Similar to metabolic acidosis, hyperventilation and respiratory alkalosis both lead to decreased P_{CO_2} and decreased H^+ secretion.

5. **The answer is C.** The NH_4^+ excreted in the urine is formed from the addition of a secreted H^+ to NH_3, which has diffused into the tubular fluid from the medullary interstitium. Once the NH_4^+ is formed, it is excreted in the urine. Increased plasma H^+ increases the secretion of H^+ by the intercalated cells and increases the production of NH_4^+ by the proximal tubule cells. Hence NH_4^+ excretion is increased. Increased proximal tubule reabsorption increases the secretion of H^+ by the proximal tubule, but excreted NH_4^+ is formed in the medullary distal nephron. Increased plasma aldosterone increases H^+ secretion. However, the increased H^+ secretion leads to a metabolic alkalosis, which decreases the production of NH_4^+. Increased filtered HCO_3^- leads to an increased H^+ secretion by the proximal tubule because of the phenomenon of glomerulotubular balance. As mentioned, NH_4^+ is formed in the more distal nephron segments. In addition, increased filtered HCO_3^- often results from increased plasma HCO_3^- concentration resulting from a metabolic alkalosis.

6. **The answer is D.** This is a difficult question because very little information is given and a definitive diagnosis cannot be made without an arterial blood sample. However, the venous plasma HCO_3^- is elevated, which indicates either a metabolic alkalosis or a compensated respiratory acidosis. If the condition were an acidosis, it might be anticipated that the plasma K^+ concentration would be increased as a result of H^+ and K^+ exchange in the cells. Since the plasma K^+ is very low, metabolic alkalosis is the most likely diagnosis. Metabolic alkalosis resulting from long-term diuretic use is a very common acid–base disorder. The purpose of the diuretic is to reduce the total body stores of Na^+ by inhibiting Na^+ reabsorption in the kidney and increasing Na^+ loss in the urine. The decrease in total body Na^+ reduces the effective circulating volume (ECV) and leads to activation of the renin–angiotensin–aldosterone system. For the body to achieve a new equilibrium at a lower ECV, the inhibiting effect of the diuretic on Na^+ reabsorption is matched by an aldosterone-stimulated increase in Na^+ reabsorption. The body comes to a new state of homeostasis with a lower ECV, which is the purpose of the diuretic. The lower ECV leads to a chronic elevation in plasma aldosterone concentration. The increased aldosterone results in increased K^+ secretion by the principal cells and an increase in H^+ secretion by the intercalated cells. The long-term increased secretion of both K^+ and H^+ lead to the hypokalemic, volume-contracted metabolic alkalosis seen in this patient.

7. **The answer is C.** Since the P_{CO_2} and the HCO_3^- are both decreased, there could either be a respiratory alkalosis with metabolic compensation or a metabolic acidosis with respiratory compensation. The only way to make the diagnosis is to determine the acid–base status, and all of the information necessary to calculate the H^+ concentration is available. Using the Henderson equation [$24 \times (P_{CO_2}/HCO_3^-)$], the H^+ concentration is 60 nmol/L. The patient is acidotic. Therefore the correct diagnosis is metabolic acidosis with respiratory compensation. Alternatively, the pH can also be estimated. If the ratio $HCO_3^-/(.03 \times P_{CO_2})$ is less than the normal of 20, the pH is decreased relative to normal. In this case the ratio is 13.3, indicating a decrease in pH.

8. **The answer is C.** The patient is acidotic because the H^+ concentration is increased. The P_{CO_2} is decreased and represents the appropriate respiratory compensation for a metabolic acidosis. The plasma HCO_3^- is decreased. Since the anion gap is increased relative to normal (10–16 mEq/L), the plasma HCO_3^- has been consumed in the buffering of exogenous acid. In this case, the acidosis is probably the result of an accidental ingestion of an acidic substance.

9. **The answer is C.** Examination of the blood gas data indicates a pH of 7.20, clearly an acidic condition. There are only two possibilities for an acidosis. The P_{CO_2} would be increased if the primary cause was respiratory, but it is decreased. The other possibility is a decreased HCO_3^- resulting from metabolic causes. Since the HCO_3^- is decreased, the cause is metabolic. The decreased P_{CO_2} is the respiratory compensation for a metabolic acidosis.

10. **The answer is C.** The patient is very acidotic, and the HCO_3^- is decreased; therefore, there is a metabolic component. In spite of the fact that the respiratory rate is very high, the P_{CO_2} is slightly elevated and indicates a respiratory acidosis. If the respiratory function is slightly improved, the patient may be able to lower the arterial P_{CO_2} to a less than normal value. However, a small decrease in P_{CO_2} to less than normal would still be insufficient to compensate for the marked metabolic acidosis.

11. **The answer is D.** The patient is acidotic because the pH is low and the H^+ concentration is high. The anion gap ($Na^+ - Cl^- - HCO_3^-$) equals 35 and is increased above normal. Thus the acidosis is due to addition of acid to the body and not the loss of HCO_3^- as a result of diarrhea. The only remaining question is the source of the acid. The creatinine is six times normal, and renal function is impaired. Recall from earlier chapters that retention of metabolic by-products is a major characteristic of renal failure. The source of the acids in the body is the result of the impaired kidney's inability to excrete titratable acids and NH_4^+ and generate new HCO_3^-. The continued production of H^+ from normal protein metabolism is simply greater than the ability of the kidney to excrete it. The body stores of HCO_3^- are consumed in the buffering of the metabolic acids, and the plasma HCO_3^- concentration is decreased. Many patients with severe renal impairment are placed on a low-protein diet to prevent just such clinical complications.

INDEX

NOTE: Page numbers with an *f* Indicate figures; those with a *t* indicate tables.